THE

PFIZER

PAPERS

The Secret Documents Exposing Big Pharma's
COVID Vaccine Crimes

By

T.J. Coles

URSA MAJOR

By the same author

Britain's Secret Wars

The Great Brexit Swindle

President Trump, Inc.

Voices for Peace (ed.)

Human Wrongs

Fire and Fury

Real Fake News

Union Jackboot (with Matthew Alford)

Manufacturing Terrorism

Privatized Planet

Your Brain in Quarantine

The War on You

Capitalism and Coronavirus

We'll Tell You What to Think

Where Does Prejudice Come From?

Biofascism

Militarizing Cancel Culture

This edition published by Ursa Major

Cover design by Jack Q. Boom

Author's Biography

T.J. Coles was a postdoctoral researcher at Plymouth University's Cognition Institute in the UK, until a cabal of staff, led by Associate Professor Jane Grant, cancelled him over his political views. No specific allegations were ever made. He was working on a device to help blind and visually impaired people and on a series of articles exposing elite child trafficking.

Undeterred, Coles continues to write for a number of publications and is the author of several books about politics and neuroscience, including *Where Does Prejudice Come From?* His latest is *Militarizing Cancel Culture* and he can be contacted via the Plymouth Institute for Peace Research.

Acknowledgements

Thanks to Laura, my wife, for help with the manuscript. Errors and shortcomings are entirely my own.

Contents

Acronyms..........8

Introduction.........10

Chapter 1.........19

Chapter 2.........27

Chapter 3.........33

Chapter 4.........40

Chapter 5.........46

Chapter 6.........52

Chapter 7.........58

Chapter 8.........64

Chapter 9.........71

Chapter 10.........78

Chapter 11.........84

Chapter 12.........91

Chapter 13.........98

Chapter 14………107

Conclusion……….114

Medical Glossary……….121

Appendix: The Nuremberg Code……….127

Endnotes………130

Index……….157

Acronyms

ADEPT Autonomous Diagnostics to Enable Prevention and Therapeutics
AEFI Adverse events following immunization
AESI Adverse event of special interest
BMJ British Medical Journal
CDC Centers for Disease Control and Prevention
CEPI Coalition for Epidemic Preparedness Innovations
CI Confidence interval
COVID Coronavirus Disease 2019
COX-I Cytochrome c oxidase I
DARPA Defense Advanced Research Projects Agency
DNA Deoxyribonucleic acid
DoD Department of Defense
EUA Emergency Use Authorization
FDA Food and Drug Administration
FOI(A) Freedom of Information (Act)
FSGS Focal segmental glomerulosclerosis
GAVI Vaccine Alliance
GCGH Grand Challenges in Global Health
GMO Genetically modified organism
HCV Hepatitis C virus
HIV Human immunodeficiency virus
IgG Immunoglobulin G
IP Internet Protocol
LNB Laboratory notebook
LNPs Lipid nanoparticles
mcg Microgram

mRNA Messenger ribonucleic acid
NPs Nanoparticles
PCR Polymerase chain reaction
PEG Polyethylene glycol
PGE2 Prostaglandin E2
PHMPT Public Health and Medical Professionals for Transparency
PREPARE PReemptive Expression of Protective Alleles and Response Elements
QCS Quality control serum
RBD Receptor-binding Domain
RCT Randomly-controlled trials
RNA Ribonucleic acid
SADS Sudden adult death syndrome
SARS-CoV-2 Severe Acute Respiratory Syndrome Coronavirus 2
SPEAC Safety Platform for Emergency Vaccines
VAERS Vaccine Adverse Event Reporting System
WHO World Health Organization

Introduction
Maddie's Story

In December 2020, Patrick and Stephanie de Garay, a middle-aged couple from Ohio, were paid by the drug giant Pfizer to enrol their three children in a COVID vaccine trial.[1]

The de Garay family went along to the Cincinnati Children's Hospital Vaccine Research Center/Vaccine Treatment and Evaluation Unit, which hosted the trial.[2]

On 20th January 2021, their daughter Maddie's life changed forever. Within 12 hours of receiving her second injection, Maddie went from being a happy, healthy, 12-year-old to being wheelchair-bound and fed through a tube.

According to her mother, Stephanie, Maddie suffered:

> ...severe abdominal pain, painful electric shocks on her spine and neck, swollen extremities, ice cold hands and feet, chest pain, tachycardia [rapid heartbeat], pins and needles in her feet that eventually led to the loss of feeling from her waist down. She had blood in her urine from 7 tests over 3 months, mysterious rashes, peeling feet, reflux, gastroparesis, vomiting, and eventually the

inability to swallow liquids or food, dizziness, passing out, convulsions, the inability to sweat, swollen lymph nodes in her armpits, urinary retention, heavy periods with clots of blood, decreased vision, tinnitus, memory loss, mixing up words, extreme fatigue, and sadly more.[3]

How many people, including children and babies, have been killed or seriously injured by Pfizer and the other drug giants as a result of their injectable products?

The media have helped Pfizer and the other companies to cover up injection injuries. But as the months go by, we are seeing, drip by drip, a growing number of injection-injured people coming forward.

Pfizer didn't want to release its clinical trial data, in part because similar stories to Maddie's would come to public attention.

Additionally, the company wanted the world to wait for 55 years before being able to analyse the data of the very product it was injecting into people.[4]

But a Texas Judge, Mark Pittman, ordered the release of the Pfizer-BioNTech papers. I have spent more than a year reading the documents released to date. I have written this book to reveal to readers what exactly is in the documents.

ABOUT THIS BOOK

This book assumes that the reader is intelligent but not an expert in biology or vaccinology. It does not shy away from complex topics. If parts seem repetitious, it is merely to remind the non-specialist reader of the meanings of certain terms.

A medical glossary and acronyms key are provided for ease of reference.

Chapter 1 is about Brook Jackson, the Ventavia whistleblower. Chapter 2 uncovers the corruption of science. Chapter 3 analyses the recent medical literature on adverse reactions to the mRNA injections. Chapter 4 charts how mRNA technology originated in the military. Chapters 5 to 14 go through the FOIA-released Pfizer documents. The Conclusion warns about our collective, mRNA future.

Interpretations of the papers are my opinions. Readers may disagree, but all claims are linked to source material so you can make up your own minds.

PROFITS BEFORE PEOPLE

Given Maddie's tragic experience, the trial would, in normal times, have been stopped with immediate effect and the vaccine candidate withdrawn.[5]

But these were not normal times. Government and big pharma said that they wanted to weigh the risks of vaccination, which they claimed were very low, with the alleged need to inoculate the world against SARS-CoV-2.

The reality is that big pharma used the pandemic as a once-in-lifetime opportunity to double their profits.[6] Five-and-a-half *billio*n people received at least one injection.[7] (There are no figures specifying which products, but Pfizer's appears to lead in the West by a long way.) Over 13 billion injections were administered to humans worldwide.[8]

Big pharma rushed an experimental product to a global population held hostage by vaccine mandates imposed by their governments. At the peak of the pandemic, Pfizer, BioNTech, and Moderna made $1,000 in profit *every second*,[9] with Pfizer charging $19.50 per dose in the US.[10]

Did profit or medical necessity dictate the perceived need for multiple boosters?

COVER-UP

When it comes to Pfizer, they refused to publish data on their clinical trials because the data, obtained in court filings, show that the company fudged the numbers to make the experimental product look more efficacious than it is. They concealed vaccine-related deaths and injuries.

Maddie de Garay's story is, sadly, one of many. By economically coercing and socially pressuring people to take a novel, for-profit injection without informed consent, governments and drug giants have perpetrated a major crime against humanity.

Yet, they are shielded from scrutiny by the propaganda system and by a prevailing cultural assumption: that vaccines were the best and indeed only option out of the pandemic, so any possible side-effects were worth the risk.

Pfizer, the for-profit health system, and local health providers covered up Maddie's life-destroying injuries.

The US uses VAERS, the Vaccine Adverse Event Reporting System. VAERS is part of the Health and Human Services department and relies on vaccine recipients voluntarily reporting their injuries and suspected injuries.

The de Garay parents wrote to Robert Frenck, Pfizer's principal investigator at the Cincinnati Children's Hospital. After reportedly ignoring them, Frenck eventually responded, explaining that doctors involved in the trial do not report to VAERS but to Pfizer. (This is consistent with documents I've seen and analysed.)

The de Garay family alleged that Dr. Frenck reported to Pfizer only Maddie's "functional abdominal pain and paresthesia," ignoring the rest.

But it was also the responsibility of Pfizer investigators to follow up on the health of their trial participants. Not a single person from Pfizer, the Food and Drug Administration, the National Institutes of Health, or the Centers for Disease Control and Prevention contacted the family to discuss what happened to Maddie.

Emails suggest that Dr. Frenck even delayed giving the family Maddie's vaccine trial tracking number.

At the time of writing, Pfizer has not honoured its obligation to pay for Maddie's potentially life-long, post-injury care. Indeed, Pfizer.com says: "0 search results for 'de garay'." The only mainstream media outlet that covered Maddie's tragedy was the right-wing Fox News.

Pfizer continued to push the government to authorise the dangerous, experimental product for nationwide distribution into the arms of millions of children.

FORCED INJECTIONS

Governments round the world forced their populations into lockdown. Once various companies had produced purported vaccinations, governments then coerced their publics into taking the injection under threat of losing their jobs—i.e., means of survival—and/or education.

They told their captive populations that getting injected was the only route out of lockdown and the only path to continued employment. This was a blatant violation of the Nuremberg Code which protects informed consent and medical freedom of choice.

Had people known about Maddie's torture, they might have been less willing to take the injection.

The World Health Organization (WHO) is a body of the United Nations. It offers health advice to sovereign states and provides health programmes to poorer countries.

Yet, the WHO has been thoroughly corrupted by money. In May 2022, the WHO published an ethics paper designed to try to justify forced injections.

It starts by arguing, without evidence, that vaccines are the best way out of a pandemic. It then goes on to compare a permanent, invasive medical procedure to cars stopping at red lights. It says that injection mandates are ethical because:

> in many parts of the world, people are required to wear seatbelts, motorists with poor visual acuity are required to wear corrective lenses, restaurant owners are required to regularly submit to food service inspections and medical assessments are required for certain jobs.[11]

CORRUPTING THE SCIENCE

How come the WHO is pushing a totalitarian policy? Of course, the answer is money.

Bill Gates is a centibillionaire who has made a significant percentage of his fortune from vaccine technology, particularly patent-protected intellectual properties on vaccine cooling technologies.

Gates told the World Economic Forum that his "philanthropy" is, in reality, a 20-to-1 return on investments, making him and his investors $200 billion over two decades.[12]

Bill Gates funds the Vaccine Alliance (GAVI) and the Coalition for Epidemic Preparedness Innovations (CEPI).

The WHO's funding is opaque and complicated. The Organization breaks its funding into "assessed contributions," "donations," and "voluntary contributions," making it hard to know exactly how much money NGOs are contributing compared to governments.[13]

An investigation by *Politico* found that GAVI and CEPI fund a significant portion of the WHO's budget. Since the start of the pandemic, GAVI, CEPI, and the Wellcome Trust donated "significantly greater amount[s] than most other official member states, including the United States and the European Commission."[14]

But Gates and his cronies also directly lobbied the governments of sovereign states, meeting US President Joe Biden, UK Prime Minister Boris Johnson, and German Chancellor Angela Merkel, and other top politicians and bodies, over 100 times to advise on pandemic management.[15]

JUSTICE FOR MADDIE?

At the time of writing, Maddie and her family remain without help. In the autumn of 2021, Dr. Frenck, concealing what happened to the girl, gave a self-congratulatory interview for an article ironically entitled, "Building Trust One Shot at a Time."

Was the medical profession more interested in prioritising safety or building trust? It's easy to build trust if you don't tell the truth about trial participant injuries.

The article says that the FDA's:

…decision to authorize the first COVID-19 vaccine for young children was based, in part, on data from clinical trials conducted by [Dr. Robert Frenck] and his team at Cincinnati Children's Hospital Medical Division.[16]

Would that decision have been made if Maddie's story had been included in the data?

Frenck described the pressure under which he felt to deliver results: "We were watching the world burn, knowing that people were counting on us for vaccine results and hoping for efficacy rates of at least 50% to 60%."[17]

Is this an admission that pressure led to biased results?

It was Pfizer, not a neutral health provider, that apparently informed Frenck that the injectable product was purportedly 95 percent effective (which, as we shall see, turned out to be a lie).

"It literally felt like a 10,000-pound weight was lifted off my shoulders ... All the work had been worth it."[18]

Maddie still bears that weight. Was it worth it for her and the thousands like her?

Chapter 1
Cover-Up

It was clear from the outset that any new injectable product purportedly designed to fight COVID was unlikely to be safe or effective, as measured by previous vaccines.

Of course, political point-scoring played a big role.

In order to look good on the world stage, Russia rolled out Sputnik V: an alleged anti-COVID vaccine. Western governments and scientific papers were right to quickly dismiss the product as having been developed too fast.[19]

Britain developed the Oxford-AstraZeneca product, which the European Union suspended because it was causing blood clots.[20] The US refused to license it.[21]

Why was the product OK for Brits but for no one else? It is likely because Pfizer, BioNTech, and Moderna successfully lobbied the US and EU countries to ensure that *their* products, and not the British one, were prioritised.

Using the media to minimise injection side-effects, the British government wanted to make as much money for AstraZeneca as possible and to stimulate a sense of national pride in the alleged vaccine.

Pfizer and the German firm BioNTech collaborated to create a novel, genetically-engineered purported vaccine, one made with mRNA, like the Moderna product.

But it soon transpired that the mRNA injections were causing fainting and heart problems in significant numbers of people. Why were they allowed to dominate the captive market but the equally dangerous Russian and British vaccines not allowed to compete?

More importantly, why did the prospective Biden administration[22] and leading scientists[23] say clearly that rushing the production of a COVID vaccine was potentially dangerous, yet as soon as they took power from the Trump administration, they promoted and indeed mandated the Pfizer and Moderna products?

In September 2020, before doing a 180, Dr. Peter Hotez said: "We don't do EUAs [Emergency Use Authorizations] for vaccines ... It's a lesser review, it's a lower-quality review, and when you're talking about vaccinating a large chunk of the American population, that's not acceptable."[24]

WHISTLEBLOWER

Capitalism works, in part, by third-party outsourcing. Instead of Pfizer's clinical trials being conducted under a centralised, public-interest authority, the structure involved myriad private clinics, hospitals, laboratories, and equipment suppliers/analysts.

This structural mess was an obvious recipe for disaster: for corner-cutting, data fudging, and adverse event under-reporting.

The pandemic-panicked culture demanded speedy and positive results. Laboratories cut safety and analytic corners to deliver those results, as one courageous whistleblower, Brook Jackson, confirmed.

Jackson's important revelations were almost completely ignored by the media and, more appallingly, by the medical profession, with the noble exception of the BMJ (formerly *British Medical Journal*), whose co-editor Dr. Peter Doshi is one of the very few influential doctors globally to speak critically of the injectable products.

A clinical auditor by profession, Jackson was regional director of Ventavia, the for-profit clinical research company based in Texas. Jackson spent her mere fortnight at Ventavia repeatedly warning and complaining to staff about poor practices.[25]

These included unblinding trial participants by leaving their details on display for medical professionals to see.[26]

According to the BMJ: "the company wasn't able to quantify the types and number of errors they were finding when examining the trial paperwork for quality control."[27]

Perhaps most serious of all, Jackson alleges that Ventavia failed to report on patients' adverse reactions to the vaccine candidates.

Jackson warned the Food and Drug Administration, which covered it up. Ventavia fired Jackson. Jackson noted (from the BMJ):

- Participants placed in a hallway after injection and not being monitored by clinical staff
- Lack of timely follow-up of patients who experienced adverse events
- Protocol deviations not being reported
- Vaccines not being stored at proper temperatures
- Mislabelled laboratory specimens, and
- Targeting of Ventavia staff for reporting these types of problems.[28]

In Pfizer's submission to the FDA requesting Emergency Use Authorization, the serious issues documented at the Ventavia trial were completely omitted.[29]

COURTS

In January 2021, Jackson took Pfizer, Ventavia, and the Ireland-based subcontractor Icon, to court under the False Claims Act.

The lawsuit alleges that the companies "concealed violations of both their clinical trial protocol and federal regulations, including falsification of clinical trial documents."[30]

The Pfizer papers analysed in this book lend weight to the allegation. The lawsuit further alleges that:

In the race to secure billions in federal funding and become the first to market, [Pfizer et al.] deliberately withheld crucial information from the United States that calls the safety and efficacy of their vaccine into question ...

Due to [Pfizer et al.'s] scheme, millions of Americans have received a misbranded vaccination which is potentially not as effective as represented. The vaccine's [FDA] authorization resulted from a deeply flawed clinical trial that violated FDA regulations.[31]

Again, the documents analysed in this book bear this out.

FRAUD

Jackson's lawsuit gives us a precise insight into how the alleged fraud was perpetrated.

The allegations outlined in the lawsuit are more specific and serious than the BMJ's rendering. Jackson claims that she witnessed:

1. The "fabrication and falsification" of participant data;
2. The enrolment of ineligible persons (including Ventavia staff);
3. Failure to obtain informed consent;
4. Not recording patients' prior COVID infections;

5. Over-diluting the vaccine concentrate;
6. Not waiting long enough for the product to thaw; and
7. "Ventavia did not report all clinical trial participants' pregnancies to Pfizer and Icon [another contractor] as required."[32]

The lawsuit alleges that Ventavia was compensated by Pfizer per patient, so it made economic sense to enrol as many patients as possible, including disqualified persons.

For people not in a high-risk category, the best immunity against COVID was natural. Point four suggests that the 95 percent efficacy rate claimed by Pfizer may have been based, in part, on some patients actually getting natural, not vaccine, immunity.

Point five suggests that maybe fewer trial participants were getting seriously injured than those in the general population because some of the trial doses had been over-diluted and the potency and thus danger of the product was diminished in the trial but not in the public roll-out.

Jackson further alleges that Ventavia did not give trial participants their second vaccine dose within the 19 to 23-day window, yet reported that they did.

This is important, because if trial participants were more likely to have adverse reactions from a second injection within 23 days, yet received their second dose later, it would make the product seem safer than it is.

On or around September 14, 2020, Ventavia discovered that randomization confirmation pages had improperly been placed in *every patient's chart*. These pages unblind the reader by revealing whether or not the patient received a placebo, and had been in place since the beginning of Ventavia's involvement in the Pfizer-BioNTech trial. Approximately 1,200 patients' charts were affected, compromising the integrity of the trial. (Emphasis added).[33]

IGNORE AND SMEAR

Jackson's story has been suppressed by state-corporate media. Her public appearances are largely confined to independent podcasts.

As more data about adverse reactions come to light in the medical literature and Jackson's star in the alternative media continues to slowly rise, hit-pieces emerge.

One of the worst is a fake website: www.brookjackson.com. The site gives the initial appearance of being Ms. Jackson's, but it soon becomes clear that it is designed to question her integrity.

IP tracking sites claim that the site is hosted by host2.westbullock.com. The latter is alleged by IP tracking services to be a datacentre and marketing company based in Lansing, Michigan.[34]

At the time of writing, lawyers for Pfizer, Icon, and Ventavia are continuing to find technicalities on which to file motions of opposition to Jackson's lawsuit, but Jackson continues to fight back.

Chapter 2
Corrupting "the Science"

Maddie de Garay's appalling injuries have not made it into any official datasets. To know the truth, we have to rely on medical professionals and editors with integrity who are willing to publish vaccine-related death and injuries in peer-reviewed journals.

In November 2020, it was widely reported that the Pfizer product was 95 percent safe and effective. But the data came from Pfizer, not from independent verification.

How did Pfizer reach its "95 percent effective" number?

Of the 43,661 trial participants, the company found just 170 individuals who tested positive for symptomatic COVID.

Of those 170, just eight had received the vaccine candidate and the remaining 162 had received a placebo.[35] Eight is 4.7 percent of 170. Rounding to five, Pfizer concluded that the jab was 95 percent effective.

In non-pandemic times, most medical professionals would consider this to be an unacceptably small sample size (170 people), especially as it drew from an acceptably larger sample (>44k).

But, panicked by pandemic propaganda and brainwashed into prioritising vaccines above other health interventions (e.g., increased vitamin intake), medical professionals went along with the scam.

The sleight-of-hand is even more evident when we put Brook Jackson's revelations about forged data and hidden patient injuries, like Maddie de Garay's, into context.

Further limiting their use, it is also important to stress that the clinical trials were not designed to assess whether the novel products could interrupt viral transmission.

BUYING THE F.D.A.

In November 2020, it was widely reported that the Pfizer product was 95 percent safe and effective.

But a closer reading demonstrates that the headlines were unchallenged, Pfizer propaganda.

For example, the *New York Times* published an article entitled: "New Pfizer Results: Coronavirus Vaccine Is Safe and 95% Effective." But the author/their editor waited until the end of the piece to reveal that Pfizer had not yet submitted safety data to the Food and Drug Administration.[36]

Two months later, NBC quoted a purported FDA document "proving" the 95 percent efficacy rate.[37]

But the document says on the front page, "Sponsor: Pfizer and BioNTech."[38] So, the document was not the FDA but Pfizer/BioNTech using the FDA as a front.

The document claims: "The proposed dosing regimen is 2 doses, 30 μg each, administered 21 days apart."

But as we shall see, the Pfizer documents show that different trial participants were given different micrograms of mRNA. Jackson alleged that some participants actually received their second dose later than 21 days (or 23 as in the Ventavia trial).

The purported FDA document says that the trials were double-blinded. But, not only did Jackson allege that unblinding had occurred, some of the Pfizer documents themselves acknowledge this.

The document also says that the placebo to vaccine candidate ratio was 1:1. But, as we shall see, some Pfizer documents mention a 4:1 ratio, meaning that some participants received more vaccine candidates than placebos. The FDA/Pfizer release does not make clear which group received which ratio.

INDEPENDENT REVIEWS?

At the end of December 2020, medical professionals reviewed clinical trial data and published findings in respected peer-reviewed journals.

Like Pfizer and the FDA, they vouched for the new product's safety and efficacy.

The triangle, it seemed, was complete: the company, the government, and independent scientists all said that the vaccine was good.

But on closer inspection, the "science" was institutionally corrupt.

There is no suggestion that any of the scientists behaved improperly.

Rather, in my opinion, being sponsored by a drug giant is inherently unethical, even if you declare the sponsor, because of the innate bias towards producing results favourable to the sponsor.

In the *New England Journal of Medicine*, bolstering the Pfizer/FDA claims, Polack et al. began their analysis by stating that "Safe and effective vaccines are needed urgently."[39]

Notice that they were not interested in finding non-vaccine interventions. Their starting point was prioritising a vaccine.

In the conflicts of interest section of the article, it not only says that the study was sponsored by Pfizer and that two individuals gave "editorial support funded by Pfizer," in the acknowledgements, more than 60 Pfizer employees/contractors are thanked.

COMMON SENSE

Dr. Peter Doshi is a rarity in the medical field.

A multi-award- and grant-winner, he is an Associate Professor of Practice, Sciences, and Health Outcomes Research at the University of Maryland-Baltimore. Doshi researches how drugs are approved, including the risks and benefits.

Doshi is a senior editor at the BMJ. He is the type who would normally go-along-to-get-along. Yet, he doesn't.

Instead, this highly-regarded medical professional did what most of his colleagues failed, refused, or were unable to do. He risked his career and reputation to use logic and basic decency to question the safety and efficacy of the new, injectable products.

In early 2021, as state-corporate media and pharma-sponsored journals were touting the brilliance of the purported vaccine, Doshi authored an opinion piece in the BMJ,[40] pointing out that the only public documents at the time were press releases and study protocols.

He observed that by early-2021, just two peer-reviewed journal articles confirmed the supposed safety and efficacy of the new products: one was Pfizer-sponsored Polack paper noted above, the other vouching for the Moderna injection was authored by scientists who own(ed) stock options in Moderna.[41]

The notorious 170 confirmed COVID cases exclude an additional 3410 suspected cases. Why weren't those suspected cases confirmed and analysed?

Doshi further notes that, of the 3410 suspected cases, 1594 occurred in the vaccine candidate group and 1816 in the placebo cohort.[42]

He estimates that vaccine candidate efficacy against developing COVID symptoms, without a positive test result, reducing the efficacy to 19 not 95 percent: "far below the 50% effectiveness threshold for authorization set by regulators."[43]

The type of test used, the PCR, can produce false-negatives. If many of the suspected cases were false-negatives, he says, it would further decrease the efficacy.

The trials did not control for non-COVID ailments that produced COVID-like symptoms, such as flu.

Excluded from the trial efficacy analyses were 371 participants due to protocol deviations on or before the seventh day following the second dose.[44]

But the numbers were not roughly even. Of the 371, 311 were from the vaccine candidate group and only 60 from the placebo group. Why the imbalance?

Appallingly, COVID patients were allowed to take pain and fever medications during the vaccine candidate trials. This means that other medicines could mask the effects of the vaccine candidate.

Not only this, but participants in the vaccine group were three to four times more likely to take such medicines than in the placebo group.[45]

Chapter 3
Injuries

In their race to bring a new product to a captive global market, Pfizer, BioNTech, and the health authorities ignored and covered up adverse events, including severe ones.

The August 2023 Pfizer papers include guidelines from mid-2021, which specifically state that people with myocarditis or pericarditis should warn their health providers of their condition before getting injected.[46]

In other words, the company, and the state-corporate media, were aware of the risks, but kept quiet about it.

The company conducted no long-term studies on side-effects because the priority of the government was to develop an anti-COVID vaccine and hope that it worked.

As we shall see, the company even failed to conduct proper follow-ups of trial participants. In the end, the people of the world were the test subjects for the new product and it took independent health professionals to report on adverse events.

STANDARD PROCEDURES NOT INCLUDED

Named after the city in Britain where the initial conferences were held, the Brighton Collaboration was established in the year 2000 by the US Centers for Disease Control and Prevention with support from the World Health Organization. The purported aim of the project is to improve vaccine safety.[47]

The Coalition for Epidemic Preparedness Innovations was founded at the World Economic Forum in 2017. CEPI's supposed aim is to "accelerate the development of vaccines and other biologic countermeasures against epidemic and pandemic threats."[48]

In 2019, CEPI and the Brighton Collaboration formed the Safety Platform for Emergency Vaccines (SPEAC, sic). In March 2020, SPEAC created a priority list of potential adverse events for COVID vaccine trials.

But in mid-2022, Fraiman et al. revealed that "the list has not been applied to serious adverse events in randomized trial data."[49]

So, the researchers took the method and randomised trial data and applied it to mRNA vaccine candidate trials. They imply that the Food and Drug Administration had used an analytical method that concealed or minimised serious adverse events in the Pfizer trial: "In contrast to the FDA analysis, we found an excess risk of SAEs [severe adverse events] in the Pfizer trial."[50]

They note that "The Pfizer trial exhibited a 36 % higher risk of serious adverse events in vaccinated participants in comparison to placebo recipients."

In general:

> "the mRNA vaccines were associated with an excess risk of serious adverse events of special interest of 12.5 per 10,000 vaccinated (95 % CI 2.1 to 22.9); risk ratio 1.43 (95 % CI 1.07 to 1.92)."

The authors say: "In both Pfizer and Moderna trials, the largest excess risk occurred amongst the Brighton category of coagulation disorders. Cardiac disorders have been of central concern for mRNA vaccines."

Pfizer limited its adverse events reporting to one month after the second dose. The authors point out that this limitation a) excludes potential long-term events and b) excluded events that occurred shortly after one month. In addition, the adverse event criteria might be higher than patients' subjective experiences.

Finally, the authors criticise the exclusion of patients who suffered multiple events.

INFLAMMATION

Severe adverse reactions following mRNA injections could be due to:

> "a proinflammatory action of the lipid nanoparticles used or the delivered mRNA (i.e., the vaccine formulation), as well as to the unique nature, expression pattern, binding

profile, and proinflammatory effects of the produced antigens - spike (S) protein and/or its subunits/peptide fragments."[51]

By April 2021, there were at least "6,605, 830, and 2,292 vaccine recipients who suffered from COVID-19-related symptoms after vaccination with BNT162b2 [Pfizer], Ad26.COV2.S [Janssen], and mRNA-1273 [Moderna]."[52]

A pro-injection article published in May 2021 noted that: "the incidence of anaphylaxis episodes attributable to the Pfizer/BioNTech vaccine occurred in roughly 1:200,000 individuals (sic)."[53]

OTHER ADVERSE EVENTS

A June 2021 study, which champions the injection, found that "from 704,003 first-doses recipients; 6536 [adverse events following immunization] were reported, of whom 65.1% had at least one neurologic AEFI (non-serious 99.6%)."[54]

By September 2021, "1.243 cases of myocarditis after vaccination with BNT162b2 Comirnaty© were registered in young adults by the Paul-Ehrlich-Institute in Germany alone."[55]

Another study from that period points out that COVID increases the risk of illnesses that are also associated with mRNA injections. The authors deduce that the risk-benefit ratio favours injection:[*]

> "Vaccination was most strongly associated with an elevated risk of myocarditis (2.7 events per 100,000 persons), lymphadenopathy (78.4 events per 100,000 persons), appendicitis (5.0 events per 100,000 persons), and herpes zoster infection (15.8 events per 100,000 persons)."[56]

A study of injection recipients in Hong Kong identified clotting (thromboembolism) as an adverse event of special interest (AESI):

> "The most frequently reported AESI among CoronaVac and BNT162b2 recipients was thromboembolism (first dose: 431 and 290 per 100,000 person-years; second dose: 385 and 266 per 100,000 person-years)."[57]

An October 2021 study part-financed by Pfizer and others, found:[†]

---

[*] Confidence intervals excluded for ease of reading, risk differences included for context.

[†] Confidence and RR intervals removed for ease of reading.

"The incidence of [adverse] events per 1 000 000 person-years during the risk vs comparison intervals for ischemic stroke was 1612 vs 1781; for appendicitis, 1179 vs 1345; and for acute myocardial infarction, 935 vs 1030. No vaccine-outcome association met the prespecified requirement for a signal. Incidence of confirmed anaphylaxis was 4.8 per million doses of BNT162b2 and 5.1 per million doses of mRNA-1273 [Moderna]."[58]

In March 2023, Yasmin and the team analysed the data of 17,636 individuals who had been injected and reported subsequent cardiovascular complications. "N =" means the number of individuals with the particular adverse event:

"Of 17,636 cardiovascular events with any mRNA vaccine, 17,192 were observed with the BNT162b2 (Pfizer-BioNTech) vaccine, 444 events with mRNA-1273 (Moderna). Thrombosis was frequently reported with any mRNA vaccine (n = 13,936), followed by stroke (n = 758), myocarditis (n = 511), myocardial infarction (n = 377), pulmonary embolism (n = 301), and arrhythmia (n = 254)."[59]

TIP OF THE ICEBERG

These are just of the severe adverse events (SAEs) suffered by hundreds of thousands of injection recipients.

A growing body of peer-reviewed literature explores SAEs. This should have been done before the novel product was forced into the arms of hundreds of millions of people.

Chapter 4
The Military Origins of the Injection

The experimental mRNA injections were developed over a thirty-year period at the US military's bioweapons centre, Fort Detrick, and particularly over the last decade at the Defense Advanced Research Projects Agency.

The mRNA-based experimental injections are killing people. Numerous countries are reporting inexplicably high, non-COVID-related excess mortality.

A percentage of excess deaths are caused by numerous, non-injection-related factors, including dementia, cancer, organ diseases, hospital backlogs, and more.[60]

Yet, these mortality statistics do not explain all deaths.

It has been speculated by some doctors outside the mainstream that, because the injection was the common denominator, it is likely that the experimental product is responsible for the unexplained parts of excess mortality.

HOW INNOVATION IS FUNDED

The US military gave the world nuclear energy, microwaves, satellites, computers, the internet, and the data economy (via post-9/11 surveillance). World War II and 9/11 gave the US Department of Defense (DoD) pretexts to develop these systems. Today, the Pentagon is behind the emerging monopolies of genetic and bio-engineering.[61]

A new generation of pandemic preparedness and pathogenic surveillance will serve as the top-down, fear-based culture that justifies a new economy of Pentagon-produced products.[62]

Messenger ribonucleic acid (mRNA) helps to synthesise proteins.[63] Proteins are essential for human immunity.[64]

The Pfizer and Moderna injections are based on mRNA technologies. They are the first to be utilised for alleged vaccines.

In the 1980s, Dr. Robert Malone (whose questioning of the injectable product led to his demonisation by the state-corporate media), discovered the processes by which mRNA can stimulate the production of proteins.[65]

At the time, the use of mRNA was too complicated and expensive.

But, decades of taxpayer-funded research, some of it in the military sector, led to the realisation of modified mRNA for purported vaccines.

Vaccinologists reasoned that modified mRNA could replicate viral spike proteins and stimulate antibody responses in humans.

FORT DETRICK

Cytochrome c oxidase is an enzyme (proteins or RNAs that convert molecules). It is found in cell mitochondria. Cytochrome c oxidase I (COX-1) is its primary subunit. Mutations of COX-1 are thought to cause certain diseases.

Prostaglandins are lipids that aid blood flow, anti-inflammation, and contribute to healing tissue.

Prostaglandin E2 (PGE2) promotes birth and is found in inflammation pathways.

Recall that SARS-CoV-2 was a respiratory disease. Fibroblasts are cells that contribute to the connection of tissues.

To give an example of early military interest: In 1998, Captain James K. Choung of the US Military Academy submitted a Master's thesis on PGE2 COX-1 mRNAs in lung fibroblasts.
(Choung's research suggests that the prostaglandin EP2 receptor suppresses mRNA levels.)[66]

Fort Detrick is notorious for producing numerous bioweapons.

In the early-2000s, similar research to that of Choung's, was conducted at Fort Detrick and involved mRNA.[67]

Since treaties came into force, the US has developed bioweapons under the cover of studying diseases for prevention.

This is known as dual-use technology. It enables governments to avoid penalties for treaty violations.

DARPA is the Pentagon's Defense Advanced Research Projects Agency.

The organisation uses taxpayer money to research and develop high-risk, high-reward technologies for military applications.

A 2013 Pentagon publication says:

> DARPA's program in Autonomous Diagnostics to Enable Prevention and Therapeutics (ADEPT) aims to accelerate immune response to bio threats with nucleic acid-encoded antigens and antibodies.[68]

This refers to potential biomedicine and electrochemical manipulation.[69]

Another report makes clear that ADEPT sought to exploit mRNA technology specifically for vaccines. In 2011, DARPA "Began in vitro testing of mRNA vaccine constructs."[70]

A.D.E.P.T. AND P.R.E.P.A.R.E.

In 2016, Dr. Kathryn A. Whitehead of Carnegie Mellon University was awarded a DARPA grant to study "Next Generation mRNA Delivery Systems with Precise Spatial and Temporal Activity" (ADEPT).[71]

Whitehead's research helped ADEPT morph into PREPARE: PReemptive Expression of Protective Alleles and Response Elements.[72]

In 2019, for instance, she presented her research at a DARPA meeting in New York.[73]

The *Bulletin of the Atomic Scientists* commented at the time: "The program might push the limits of what is allowable under international security treaties."[74]

In 2019, shortly before SARS-CoV-2 was detected, Fort Detrick's US Army Medical Research and Development Command published a report on modified mRNA vaccines for Lassa virus: a haemorrhagic, zoonotic disease found mainly in West Africa.

The report claimed to have successfully vaccinated guinea pigs.[75]

Recall the above-mentioned military research into mRNA vaccines for the Lassa virus. Other PREPARE research included the following:

> A team led by the Georgia Institute of Technology, under principal investigator Dr. Phil Santangelo, aims to develop novel gene therapies to enable protection against a wide range of influenza strains by delivering mRNA-encoded programmable gene modulators and programmable antivirals to the lungs to boost host defenses and/or immediately halt viral replication.[76]

At the time of their creation, the Pfizer and Moderna injections were the only ones that utilised mRNA technology. DARPA casually mentions "Moderna as a contracted performer on the ADEPT program, to [use] some of the first experimental vaccines based on [mRNA]."[77]

In other words, Moderna was handed a huge taxpayer-funded military subsidy to develop an experimental product from which Pfizer also benefited.

Chapter 5
Prevent COVID, Not "Reduce Symptoms"

The release of the documents was bad news for the various US health departments and agencies, as well as for Pfizer and the injection industry more generally.

Pfizer's criminal record was already well-documented, long before SARS-CoV-2.

PFIZER: A CRIMINAL ORGANIZATION

In 2009, the Department of Justice (DoJ) wrote: "[Pfizer] agreed to pay $2.3 billion, the largest health care fraud settlement in the history of the Department of Justice, to resolve criminal and civil liability arising from the illegal promotion of certain pharmaceutical products."[78]

Pfizer misbranded its anti-inflammatory drug, Bextra, "with the intent to defraud or mislead."

The DoJ added: "The company will pay a criminal fine of $1.195 billion, the largest criminal fine ever imposed in the United States for any matter. Pharmacia & Upjohn [Pfizer] will also forfeit $105 million, for a total criminal resolution of $1.3 billion."[79]

Pfizer illegally promoted three other drugs, "Geodon, an anti-psychotic drug; Zyvox, an antibiotic; and Lyrica, an anti-epileptic drug – and caused false claims to be submitted to government health care programs for uses that were not medically accepted indications and therefore not covered by those programs."[80]

A civil settlement also revealed that Pfizer had been paying "kickbacks" to health professionals to promote its products.[81]

Barely a year goes by–literally–without Pfizer and its associates and subsidiaries being sued in the US alone for consumer protection, environmental, price, and wage violations.

The company and its spinoffs have been fined a total of $10 billion in the US alone since the year 2000.[82]

Yet, hundreds of millions of people have trusted the repeat offender with an experimental injection.

FLEEING THE SINKING SHIP

In August 2021, the Biden administration pressured the FDA to approve both the injections and so-called boosters.

In addition, Biden's administration wanted to lessen the FDA's oversight and shift responsibility to the Centers for Disease Control and Prevention, whose Foundation is openly funded by big pharma, including Pfizer.[83]

In response, the FDA's Marion Gruber and Philip Krause announced their intention to resign.[84] Their honourable decision was reflected by neither Pfizer's CEO Albert Bourla nor Dr. Anthony Fauci, the Trump-Biden administrations' Chief Medical Advisor and Director of the National Institute of Allergy and Infectious Diseases Director.

With the documents being released by court-order, Bourla the CEO of the criminal corporation, began to publicly distance himself from the injection.

Speaking to the *Washington Post* in a video upload, Bourla said that his decision to allow the never-before-used mRNA technology was based on his "instinct."[85]
Bourla distanced himself from the product by reiterating in the interview that his scientists convinced him that the technology was safe and effective.

Fauci is the other high-profile figure leaping headfirst off the "vaccine" bus. While refusing to put a date on his retirement, he told ABC: "I'd love to spend more time with my wife and family."[86]

FIGHTING FOR FREEDOM OF INFORMATION

In August 2021, the FDA approved the Pfizer-BioNTech "Comirnaty" product (BNT162b2) to be injected into people aged 16 and over.

Public Health and Medical Professionals for Transparency (PHMPT) is an organisation consisting of hundreds of recognised doctors, including Peter Doshi, senior editor of the *British Medical Journal* (BMJ).

The PHMPT filed a Freedom of Information Act request with the FDA[87] to obtain the safety data that Pfizer had supplied for its BNT162b2 reviews and trials. Sensibly, the FOIA was filed in Texas, where Republican judges are more likely to be "vaccine" sceptical and sympathetic to the interests of PHMPT.

The Justice Department, which represented the FDA, said that it would take 55 years to process the request.[88] To paraphrase a popular meme: Nothing says "trust the science" like a 55 year wait for data.

In January 2022, the Trump-appointed Northern Texas District Judge, Mark Pittman, ruled that: "The FDA shall produce the remaining documents at a rate of 55,000 pages every 30 days, with the first production being due on or before March 1, 2022, until production is complete."[89]

Presumably recognising the unfolding PR disaster, the FDA-Pfizer never challenged the District Judge's decision in a higher court and proceeded to comply, redacting crucial information such as the ratio of administered doses to deaths/injuries.[90]

CHANGING THE DEFINITION OF "VACCINE"

In late-2020/early-'21, politicians, health officials, and state-corporate media told us to "get vaccinated" to protect ourselves and others. They gave us the impression that the injection would get us "back to normal," implying that the jab protects against infection, prevents transmission, and will lead to herd immunity.

When this failed, the same people told us, starting around mid-'21, that we must get jabbed because the injections reduce "severe infection" and hospitalisation.

Indeed, online dictionaries (Merriam-Webster in this case) have changed their definitions. Until early-2021, "vaccine" meant a product that "produce[s] or artificially increase[s] immunity to a particular disease."[91]

It now apparently means a product that "stimulate[s] the body's immune response against a specific infectious agent or disease."[92]

There is a difference between increasingly and stimulating because stimulating does not necessarily mean increasing.

"PREVENT" COVID, NOT REDUCE SYMPTOMS

The first batch of Pfizer documents, released in March 2022, confirm that Pfizer originally planned for the injectable product to be an actual vaccine, as per the pre-2021 definition: that it would prevent disease, not merely reduce severe symptoms.

An nonclinical overview states: "BNT162b2 … is an investigational vaccine intended to prevent COVID-19," the disease caused by SARS-CoV-2 and, subsequently, its variants.[93]

Prevent, no less.

Those hoping to sue Pfizer and/or the Food and Drug Administration (FDA) might now argue that they were injected under the potentially fraudulent claim that the product could "prevent" disease.

The documents are important because, to date, over 5 billion people or 66 percent of the global population have been injected with one or more of a variety of alleged vaccines,[94] many of them using experimental mRNA nanotechnology in a first for the human species.

Neither Statista nor Our World in Data (two seemingly reliable sources) has information on how many Pfizer injections have been administered in certain countries (e.g., Australia), though they have data for European Union member states and the USA.

Some 360 million Pfizer doses have been given to Americans compared to 232 million Moderna doses.[95]

Chapter 6
Pfizer Used a Controversial Ratio Method

In April 2021, the US Food and Drug Administration (FDA) published a confidential Biologics License Application guide for clinical study data reviewers. The guide was for professionals analysing the results of large-scale tests of the Pfizer-BioNTech vaccine candidates.

Perhaps the most blatant breach of basic clinical trial protocol was the unblinding of the safety and analysis team for Phases II and III: phases which, as we shall see, were themselves tampered with.

UNBLINDING

The document says that the first 360 participants in Phases II/III were analysed "by unblinded team" (sic).[96]

Pre-COVID papers note, by contrast: "The gold standard clinical trial design is the double-blind, randomized, controlled trial. No standard practice exists for the 'unblinding' of trial participants."[97]

> 1) By April 2021, the Guide had been amended 12 times. Some of the amendments

were added after trials had already begun, meaning that some clinical methods were altered mid-trial.

2) Doses of between 20-μg and 50-μg were administered, but it is unclear whether the data were extrapolated, meaning that perhaps dose levels were mixed up, and thus efficacy hard to determine.

3) Ordinarily,[98] vaccine trials are conducted in Phases (I, II, III, VI). But the FDA originally called the Pfizer trial *Stages* before renaming them Phases in line with common practice. This would suggest that the FDA trial designers knew that their methods did not constitute Phases in the traditional sense and renamed them as not to draw attention to the flawed methods being used.

4) The BNT162b2 vaccine candidate was given to participants "who originally received placebo," meaning that it is not clear if their samples were added to the data, and if so whether BNT162b2 or their natural immunity had the given effect. A second bullet point says that some were given the BNT162b2 after the surveillance period, implying that those mentioned in the first bullet point were not.

5) In July 2020 the chronology was altered: Stages/Phases were "Renamed Stage 1 to Phase 1, removed Stage 2, and renamed Stage 3 to Phase 2/3."

6) Also in that month, patients with prior COVID-19 diagnoses were later excluded

from the trials, meaning that potentially, initial natural immunity got mixed into the "vaccine" data.

7) Time periods were also a hodgepodge. First, the design of Phase II/III (which according to the above actually skipped Phase II, which wasn't even a Phase but a Stage) did not include analysis of COVID cases 14 days after the second dose. This criterion, which one would think rather crucial, was added as late as October 2020. Second, in addition to the 14 days, a one-week period was later added. Ergo, we do not know for absolutely certain who contracted what or when or whether the BNT162b2 or natural immunity played a role.

8) The definition of symptoms was altered so that by October 2020 (five months into the trials), people who had two symptoms over a 4-day period were reported as having a single illness, meaning that the data could be rigged to imply that the "vaccine" reduced symptoms.

9) Clinical trials typically design follow-up periods. If patients are not survielled post-vaccine, analysts cannot tell if the vaccine worked. But intensive nasal swabbing (post-vaccine) was not originally included in the assessments.

10) Patients with higher risks of contracting SARS-CoV-2 (e.g., immunocompromised people, "criterion 4") were initially excluded

from surveillance "Because of a formatting error."

RATIOS: 4:1 NOT 1:1

Even if we ignore all of the above brazen violations of vaccine trial protocol, one of the major revelations of the document is confirmation that the vaccine candidate to placebo ratio was inverted, compared to other trials.

It is typical to give one drug/vaccine candidate at a ratio of one placebo. This way, it is easy to tell who has been helped by the given product and who has not. Depending on what the trial aims to determine, if symptoms are reduced and/or illness prevented more than statistical coincide in the candidate group, but not in the placebo group, the candidate can be said to be potentially effective and it will move into the next trial Phase.

It is normal to give one placebo for every product candidate. If there are 100 participants, 50 will get the placebo. This is called a 1:1 ratio. Less common is the 4:1 ratio, which has been critiqued by clinical practitioners and analysts.

Where the 4:1 ratio is used however, it is typically used in trials with higher numbers of participants. The FDA recommended the opposite: that the 4:1 ratio be used in the initial "Phase I" trial with fewer participants and the normal 1:1 ratio used in "Phase II/III": the major study of over 40k participants.

In May 2020, Pfizer publicly reported: "The dose level escalation portion (Stage 1) of the Phase 1/2 trial in the U.S. will enroll up to 360 healthy subjects into two age cohorts (18-55 and 65-85 years of age)."[99]

But the confidential FDA documents revealed that the 4:1 ratio was used.

BREAKING FROM CONVENTION

A 2011 paper reviewed the notion that trials will be "more attractive" to participants and clinicians if they include outcome-adaptive methods.

This means that if the given product does well in initial trials, more participants can be given the drug and fewer given the placebo. This is not science but marketing. As the authors note: "With no differential patient accrual rates because of the trial design, we find no benefits to outcome-adaptive randomization over 1:1 randomization, and we recommend the latter."[100]

If clinicians feel compelled to include outcome-adaptive methods, the authors recommend being limited to 2:1.

A 2014 anti-epileptic drug study (also of a Pfizer product) featured 161 participants with a 4:1 randomisation ratio. The study itself acknowledges: "unequal (4:1) randomization resulted in a small 150 mg/d [i.e., placebo] group, and results should be interpreted with caution."[101]

But no such cautious interpretation was afforded the Stage or "Phase I," Pfizer/BioNTech trial.

A 2015 study notes: "But many RCTs [randomly-controlled trials] use unequal allocation schemes (e.g., 2:1 or 3:1), which assign more patients to the experimental intervention."[102]

Notice that this one does not even include 4:1 because it is so comparatively rare. Recall that this study was pre-COVID, even here the authors cautioned that outcome-adaptive methods result in "frequent discordance between effect sizes in phase 3 studies and those in phase 2."[103]

Even worse, in the Pfizer study, "Phase" II was lumped with III.

Amazingly, the authors of the study critical of 4:1 ratios note that licensing success for outcome-adaptive trials is even less than the typical 50 percent that make it to Phase III.

Citing some hypothetical trial, the authors note that outcome-adaptive trials can create a sleight-of-hand that artificially boosts the efficacy percentage. Because of statistical reduction, "their probability of being allocated to the arm that is believed to be superior is 80% rather than 50%."[104]

Chapter 7
Pfizer Secretly Knew That It Would Push Three Shots

Documents from April 2021 show that the company was planning for a three-dose schedule while telling the world that two doses were safe and effective.

ONE, TWO, THREE...

In the last paragraph of page 23 of the April 2021 BNT162b2 "Clinical Overview," it is stated that a "subset" of Phase 3 participants would receive a third BNT162b2 injection or prototype between 5 to 7 months after their second dose.[105]

But there are several problems:

> 1) Phase 3 was still "ongoing," according to the documents, when they decided to test dose No. 3 So, how could they a) say that the jab was safe and effective with trials still "ongoing" and b) launch a third dose schedule in the middle of analysing dose 2?
>
> 2) The term "Phase 3" in this context is meaningless because, as we documented in the previous instalment, Pfizer/the FDA arbitrarily mixed elements of Phase 2 with 3

(which they originally called Stages), so reviewing the data we don't know who had what or when, or in what context.

3) As we shall see, Pfizer had already announced to the world that the two-dose schedule was effective, so why were they considering a third dose?

4) The "subset" of third dose trial participants included ages between 18 and 55: i.e., people unlikely to get seriously ill from a disease that mostly killed and hospitalised very elderly people.

5) The third dose was given with a 1:1 randomisation, yet as we documented in the previous chapter, the first two doses of Phase 2 (again, whatever that means in practice) were randomised with placebos at a 4:1 ratio, artificially inflating the apparent efficacy of the jab in a method that many clinicians have dubbed undesirable. (They favour the more logical and traditional 1:1 ratio: one placebo for every vaccine or product.)

6) The subset participants were planned to be COVID-naive, meaning that they had not had the infection before. Yet as we noted in the previous chapter, some of the large-scale participants for doses 1 and 2 had been diagnosed with COVID and others had not. In other words, the cohorts were a mess with statistical crossover that does not appear to have been extrapolated in the documents released so far.

7) The public were told they'd need a third injection even though the recipients of the third dose had not been evaluated in terms of which "vaccine" candidate they were given in relation to what dosage had been administered.

From the document:

> Phase 1 participants who were randomized to either BNT162b1 or BNT162b2 at dose levels of 10, 20, or 30 µg are being offered booster vaccination with BNT162b2 at 30 µg, approximately 6 to 12 months after their second dose of BNT162b1 or BNT162b2.[106]

BOURLA: "LIMITED PROTECTION"

But what are the doses for the third "booster" being given to the public? Where are the trial data?

At a World Economic Forum gathering, the centibillionaire vaccine promoter, Bill Gates, made a shocking revelation on which alternative and independent researchers picked up, but which the mainstream state-corporate media, unsurprisingly, ignored.

Gates said that future "vaccines" should provide long-term protection and prevent disease. (Err... isn't that the definition of vaccine?)

He opined without evidence that the mRNA COVID jabs had saved "millions of lives," but then added: "they don't have much in the way of duration and they're not good at infection-blocking."[107]

Gates bolstered Pfizer CEO Albert Bourla's admission from January, which was again predictably ignored by the state-corporate media that are in the pocket of Pfizer.

Bourla stumbled and said: "We know that the three, the two doses [Freudian slip?] of the vaccine offer very limited protection. The three doses, the booster, offer reasonable protection."[108] *Reasonable*? I thought that two doses were 95 percent efficacious, not that three doses were "reasonably" efficacious.

On 1st April 2021, Bourla's company claimed that two doses "Confirm High Efficacy and [Have] No Serious Safety Concerns Through Up to Six Months." The same press release claimed 95 percent effectiveness in preventing severe disease.[109]

Two weeks later, Bourla said that, actually, a third dose was likely needed. [110]

In other words, people were getting jabbed thinking they were safe from COVID and that their immunity would last at least six months. This is not only false advertising, it is gross negligence.

WHAT VACCINE REQUIRES FOUR DOSES?

Until COVID, very few vaccine schedules involved three or more doses.

A four-dose schedule of hepatitis B vaccines was limited to patients with chronic renal failure.[111]

An experiment in Sweden and the US in 1999 saw over 200 infants given three and four-dose schedules. But the schedules did not contain a single vaccine, like the alleged COVID vaccine. They contained diphtheria, tetanus and pertussis toxoids, inactivated poliovirus, and a Haemophilus influenza type-B.[112]

A five-dose nasal vaccine for the Rotarix trialled on Indian infants demonstrated no difference relative to the three-dose schedule.[113]

For the human papillomavirus vaccine, two doses were given to adolescent girls and assumed to afford protection for *two decades*, with a third assumed to generate *life-long protection*.[114]

This is very different to the COVID "booster" every few months.

A three- to four-dose schedule of Hantaan virus vaccine was administered to trial participants in late-2020, resulting in adverse events in around 30 percent of patients.[115]

It was only after the COVID jabs arrived on the scene that fourth-dose schedules started to become common (e.g., for tick-borne encephalitis).[116]

In late-2021, a study in *The Lancet* was published involving several thousand people--average age *below* the typical COVID death cohort--who had received three injections from different or the same products (homologous and heterologous). The results claimed that three injections was best:

> the immunogenicity of homologous or heterologous third dose boost with all tested vaccines was superior to control [i.e., placebo

or two-dose] regardless of which vaccine had been received in the initial course.[117]

But this contradicts Pfizer's claim: that two doses are good for 6 months.

UNAUTHORIZED

If *The Lancet* study designers could think to include a third dose after two had been completed and assessed, why couldn't the designers of the Pfizer trial? Is it because they wanted to rush a garbage and potentially dangerous product to market as soon as possible in order to profit from an audience made captive by injection mandates?

Pfizer began a third dose study while continuing trials of the second dose. Despite this, it saw fit to declare that two doses were effective for 6 months. No sooner had they made the claim, CEO Bourla stated that three doses might be needed, even though it would have taken Pfizer until at least October 2021 to discern that information from trial participants, yet the FDA authorised the third dose in September, with trial data still pending.

Chapter 8
Pfizer Covered Up Patient Deaths

Documents suggest that after several trial participants died--following injection with the experimental product--Pfizer covered up their deaths by attributing them to natural causes, existing conditions, and even by mere assumption that the given death was not triggered by the injection.

Before bringing the injectable product to market, supposedly to tackle the COVID pandemic, Pfizer held clinical trials, as per normal when developing new drugs and vaccines.

ABNORMAL PROCEDURES

But as documented, the trials did not meet normal clinical standards: Phases were initially called Stages before being chronologically mixed; cohorts were over-weighted for young and middle-aged people when in fact elderly are most at risk of death from/with COVID; prior COVID infections (i.e., natural immunity), were not always counted for; too few placebos were administered; and Pfizer knew that a third dose of the professed vaccine would be needed while marketing the product as two-dose "safe and effective."

We already know that in brazen violation of trial protocol, the participants of the initial Stage (later renamed Phase) were unblinded.

The stratification of data is a complete mess. For instance, the key to one chart says:[118] "* = subjects who originally received placebo and then received BNT162b2 [the vaccine candidate] after unblinding, ∞ = subjects who originally received BNT162b2."

So, unblinded participants (some initially blinded) received both a placebo and BNT162b2, but we don't know during what Phase, and others just received BNT162b2 but remained blinded?

MIXING UP THE PATIENTS

In other violations, placebo and BNT162b2 recipients were mixed. So, in other documents when "placebo" recipients were listed as having died, it could mean that BNT162b2 recipients had also died because their initial designation as placebo patient was recorded.

The court-ordered release of a 3.6k-plus page PDF contained in the zip file, dedicates three pages to deceased participants. It was published internal to Pfizer-FDA in April 2021.

Fifteen participants mentioned in the document died after receiving at least one dose of BNT162b2, yet as we shall see, Pfizer does not attribute any death to the injection.

Unlike a second document examined below, this one does not make clear which patients died after being administered the placebo compared to the

BNT162b2. Unlike the second document, it does not mention injection dosage.

Thirty-nine patients died, at least six of whom died from events definitely unrelated to COVID and/or the injection: cancer, road accidents, and a drug overdose. Other causes of death are less clear-cut, such as sepsis and arteriosclerosis.

As noted above, the key to the chart mentions "unblinding" but it is not clear if it refers to unblinded placebo and/or BNT162b2.

PATIENT DEATHS

Of the possible BNT162b2-related deaths of the remaining 15 participants who received at least one dose, symptoms/causes of death included: COVID, chronic pulmonary obstructive disease, and heart attack—myocarditis being a now well-established side-effect.

One cause of death was listed as "unevaluable." But I thought that all participant deaths in clinical trials were supposed to be evaluated?

The second latest, court-ordered release is another 3.6k-plus page document[119] published internally in November 2020. It details adverse reactions to the vaccine candidate BNT162b2 during the clinical "trials."

A common pattern emerges: Pfizer and the FDA minimise the deaths and do not attribute them to BNT162b2. Instead, they highlight natural causes, existing conditions, and mere assumption.

Part of the cover-up involved nonsensical criteria. We were told that COVID kills people because existing conditions such as obesity, plus infection with COVID, tips the body over the edge into death.

Yet, Pfizer says that where participants had existing conditions, like obesity, adverse reactions to the BNT162b2 were not the cause/trigger of death. In other words, it's one standard for COVID deaths and another for possible injection-related deaths.

Surely by the same standard, the deaths of patients with existing conditions who died following injection were likely triggered by the injection? Yet, in case after case, Pfizer says no. They don't actually study the given death, they accept the word of the given principal investigator.

Had the deaths been listed as caused/triggered by the injection, the product would have been withdrawn before getting emergency use authorisation.

ANOTHER DOCUMENT, MORE DEATHS

The following victims are from the second document, so it is not clear if some are the same as the fifteen BNT162b2-injected people (noted above) who died. The second document suggests even more deaths in addition to the 15.

One woman, 56, was given a two-dose schedule of 30 μg, ending August 2020. She died of cardiac arrest and cerebral edema (brain swelling) in October.

Pfizer/FDA says:

It was unknown if an autopsy was performed. In the opinion of the investigator, there was no reasonable possibility that the cardiac arrest was related to the study intervention or clinical trial procedures, as the death occurred 2 months after receiving Dose 2.

They don't know if an autopsy was conducted, yet the unnamed investigator sees fit to deny any link to the injection?

A man, 60, died in September 2020, three days after receiving a single 30 µg dose of BNT162b2. The man was obese and died of/with arteriosclerosis (a build-up of fat in the veins. We know the injection can cause clotting).

"According to the medical examiner, the probable cause of death was progression of atherosclerotic disease," says the document. "Relevant tests were unknown. Autopsy results were not available at the time of this report."

Tests unknown, autopsy report not available: yet the death definitely had nothing to do with the injection?

MORE DOCUMENTS, FEWER DETAILS

The Pfizer zip document reveals more victims not mentioned in the above report, yet it does not go into detail the way in which the above had done.

The zip document gives almost no information about patients, except that the "onset" of one death was 26 August. Interestingly, the patient was assigned a "toxicity grade." Some were rated 1, but this patient was graded 4. Cause of death was "undetermined."

Naysayers would point to the fact that the patient had the same ID as one who was given a *placebo* and also died on the same date, suggesting that they are the same person. Yet, the document says: "Vaccine dose/subject," not *placebo*, suggesting that actually these are two different people.

However, as we saw above, some participants might have been recorded in the placebo group and later given one dose of BNT162b2. Do the Pfizer data conflate placebo and vaccine deaths?

Another death of an individual listed as having had a "vaccine dose" was attributed to a "sudden cardiac" event. Their toxicity grade was also level 4 and they died on 19 October. Their participant ID is different to another 19th October death. The latter was given a placebo.

To summarise:

- None of the deaths were attributed by Pfizer-FDA to BNT162b2.

- The company and FDA covered up possible links by not investigating causes of death, even where autopsies were not available.

- Myocarditis and cardiac arrest deaths post-injection were not attributed to BNT162b2.

- Victims have been mixed up: There were deaths of apparently different individuals on the same day, or were they the same people?

- There was a seeming conflation of placebo and BNT162b2 participants.

- Details were provided for some participants but not others. Toxicity grades (of what?) were assigned to participants only in one of the two documents.

- High toxicity levels correlate with mortality as opposed to severe or mild BNT162b2 injury.

Chapter 9
Pfizer Calls It a "Product," Not a Vaccine

Explosive revelations that should have made headline news have been predictably ignored by legacy media. They include:

* Hundreds of potentially serious side-effects.[120]

* More children having severe adverse injection reactions than needing oxygen for COVID.[121]

* Increased myocarditis in young people.[122]

* Causes of death in trial participants not investigated (as documented in this book).

* An increase in spontaneous abortions and miscarriages in age groups not seriously at risk of dying from/with COVID (the *words* of the study deny this but the *numbers* support it).[123]

* Women and girls getting irregular periods.[124]

VACCINE OR "PRODUCT"?

Jacqueline O'Shaughnessy, Acting Chief Scientist of the US Food and Drug Administration (FDA), wrote to Pfizer's Regulatory Affairs Manager for Vaccines, Gosia Mineo.

O'Shaughnessy reminded Mineo that, as early as March 2020, the US Secretary of Health and Human Services "declared that circumstances exist justifying the authorization of emergency use of drugs and biological products during the COVID-19 pandemic."[125]

Notice that it says "products," as if they knew that a real *vaccine* could not be developed so fast.

In November 2020, Pfizer and BioNTech sponsored an FDA briefing paper on their new product. The FDA repeated Pfizer's fudged data.[126] As noted, the trial phases were mixed up, the placebo to vaccine ratio was at times 4:1 instead of the normal 1:1, and some of the participants unblinded.

Note the parsed phrases of the conclusion:

> based on the totality of scientific evidence available, it is reasonable to believe that the Pfizer-BioNTech COVID-19 Vaccine may be effective in preventing COVID-19 in individuals 16 years of age and older...[127]

I thought that science was based on evidence, not "belief." I thought that we were told that the injection was effective, not that it "may be effective."

REMOVING REFERENCES TO DOSE NUMBERS

Another O'Shaughnessy letter re-authorising the injection acknowledges that when the Pfizer-BioNTech product was granted Emergency Use Authorization (EUA) in December 2020, the FDA had "removed reference to the number of doses per vial after dilution."

In June 2022, the FDA authorised the injection for 6 month to four-year-olds, despite US Centers for Disease Control and Prevention data suggesting that fewer than 200 infants aged one to four have died of/with COVID in the US to date.[128]

The letter dated July 2022 re-authorised the injection and repeats the statement: "it is reasonable to believe that Pfizer-BioNTech COVID−19 Vaccine may be effective in preventing COVID-19."

Again, we were told that the injection was over 90 percent "safe and effective," not that vaccinologists "reasonably believed" that it "may be effective."

The re-authorisations occurred with little or no media coverage.

In February 2022, the FDA requested that Pfizer-BioNTech initiate a "rolling submission" for EUA. Pfizer told the public in its press release that by that date, one million American children aged four and under had tested positive for COVID.

They didn't mention that, of those, fewer than 200 had died (see above).

Pfizer also claimed that, by January 2023, "children under 4 accounted for 3.2% of the total hospitalizations due to COVID-19."[129]

They didn't mention that more children were having severe adverse injection reactions globally than those who needed ventilation for COVID.[130]

Pfizer also failed to note that, due to reliance on flawed algorithms, the CDC's COVID-19 Data Tracker had overestimated[131] COVID-related child deaths by over 400.

SUDDEN DEATH

Indicative of the lack of media interest in "sudden adult death syndrome," also known as "sudden arrhythmic" or "arrhythmia death syndrome" (SADS), the *New York Times* archive contains a total of three references for the three variations of the phrase from articles published between January 1980 and August 2022.[132]

Indeed, a journal dedicated to cardiology—presumably talking about UK cases—found just 453 SADS deaths between 1994 and 2003.[133]

One high-profile case was that of footballer Cormac McAnallen, who died of SADS in 2004.[134]

A recent freedom of information request filed for England and Wales revealed 302 SADS-related deaths between 2016 and '20.[135]

In June 2021, Joan Bakewell asked her fellow peers in the British House of Lords:

To ask Her Majesty's Government what assessment they make of avoidable deaths from Sudden Adult Death Syndrome in the United Kingdom each year and what steps they are taking to introduce screening to reduce such deaths, in particular for those involved in sporting activities.[136]

Death in athletes is more noticeable than in the general population, because ordinary people die in obscurity, whereas sportspeople frequently perish in full public view often on the grounds.

Joanna Penn replied with a claim that in 2019 alone (i.e., before the injection) there were 1,511 SADS deaths in the UK. Why did she say this and what were her sources? The claim is a massive, unfounded exaggeration perhaps designed to make SADS look quite normal to disguise the effects of what actually might be caused by the injection.[137]

This coincides with sudden, increased media interest in SADS.

STILL SPREADING

We have focused on the July re-authorisation, because the Pfizer papers seem to reveal little of interest and appears to be mostly uninterpreted patient data.

We are seeing the futility of the injection for preventing infection and spread.

Initially, Pfizer CEO Albert Bourla said that he had not been injected because other people were a priority;[138] as if there weren't enough doses for everyone in the West.

When the company realised that this was terrible PR, Bourla got the jab, or at least said he did. This is the same man who initially told us that the injection was nearly 100 percent safe and effective.

On 15th August, Bourla issued the following statement:

> I would like to inform the public that I have tested positive for COVID-19. I am grateful to have received four doses of the Pfizer-BioNTech vaccine and I am feeling well while experiencing very mild symptoms. I have started a course of PAXLOVID™ (nirmatrelvir [PF-07321332] tablets and ritonavir tablets), I am isolating in place as well as following all public health precautions.[139]

As people were being demonised for taking the anti-parasitic Ivermectin for COVID, media lied and gave the impression that Ivermectin is exclusively a horse de-wormer.

Now, Bourla says that he is taking the unlicensed Paxlovid, which is only approved by the FDA under EUA.

Many argue that Paxlovid has the same protease inhibitor effects as Ivermectin and that Pfizer merely stole the design of the off-patent anti-parasitic and marketed their expensive own brand: or "Pfizermectin," as some have dubbed the drug.

Chapter 10
Pfizreal: A Laboratory

In January 2021, the Israeli government signed an extraordinary collaboration agreement in which Pfizer used Israel as "a sort of laboratory" (Chief Scientific Officer Philip Dormitzer),[140] in which the vaccine candidate, which tellingly is described as a "product" in the agreement, was to be compared with natural immunity.

To quote the document:

> the Parties agree that it would be highly beneficial from a public health perspective to track pandemic data in accordance with vaccination compliance in a Real-World context to evaluate whether herd immunity protection is observed during the Product vaccination program rollout.[141]

The entire indemnification paragraphs are redacted.

ONE GIANT HUMAN EXPERIMENT

A critic of the project, Tehilla Shwartz Altshuler of the Israel Democracy Institute, describes it as "one of the ... widest medical experiments on humans at the 21st century."[142]

In August, a Zoom meeting of Israeli health officials was leaked. In the meeting, the health officials discussed long-term and serious adverse events from the injection.

They "identified new [neurological] side effects not listed in the consumers' leaflet, such as dizziness, tinnitus, hypoesthesia, [and] paraesthesia" (i.e., numbness and localised paralysis).[143]

In addition, the duration of adverse events was longer than those reported in the official Pfizer data. The leaflet said that side effects would typically last less than a week. But in half of cases recorded by the Israeli doctors, duration was six months.

In terms of neurological events, 65 percent of sufferers experienced symptoms lasting longer than one month.

Back pain, including in children, was another unexpected adverse event.

EXCESS MORTALITY

The leak comes at a time when European countries are reporting unexplained rises in excess mortality (i.e., death rates higher than average).

Pfizer told us that the injection was "safe and effective." It is easy to say that something is "safe and effective" when safety and efficacy are not defined: as indeed they were not in the clinical trials.

But over the last couple of years, data have emerged suggesting that the injection is neither effective (i.e., waning immunity, does not prevent infection) nor safe.

How can a vaccine candidate be safe when the normal decade of development, including pharmacovigilance, was shrunk to a few months, in the case of the rushed jab?

According to data drawn from the UK Office for Health Improvement and Disparities, non-heatwave related summer deaths in 2022 were 3,665 above the average (28k deaths in total), of which COVID contributed to 909. This means that 2,756 more people died in the summer of 2022 than expected compared to previous years.[144]

Main causes were: Ischaemic heart disease (>1.9k excess), heart failure (>1.9k excess), diabetes (>1.7k excess), diseases of the urinary system (882 excess), cerebrovascular diseases (679 excess), acute respiratory infections (430 excess), chronic lower respiratory (368 excess), and cancer (210 excess).

Cancer can be explained by delayed treatments due to health service backlogs. Diabetes can be explained by people eating and drinking more during lockdown. But what about the staggeringly high increase in heart disease and failure?

Some deaths can be attributed to long COVID, delayed hospital treatment, and lockdown stress (e.g., lack of exercise, anxiety, overeating, etc.), but the major change between 2022 and previous years is that most British people have been double, and some even triple, jabbed.

KIDNEY INJURIES

It is interesting to note urinary infection as one of the causes of excess mortality because medical journals have been reporting cases of post-injection kidney disease.

Interstitial nephritis is a condition in which the kidney's tubules are inflamed. The condition reduces the organ's ability to filter waste and fluid. Czerlau and the team found that five of their patients—they don't reveal the sample size, which is odd—experienced acute interstitial nephritis after injection.[145]

One of the patients had existing nephropathy (kidney deterioration) and four did not.

High serum creatinine (SC) levels can suggest that kidneys are in distress. The SC values of Patient 1's kidneys prior to injection were 76.5 μmol/L. After injection, they had jumped to 355 μmol/L. Patient 2's values could not be compared due to lack of prior data.

Patient 3 already had nephropathy. Their values ballooned from 167 μmol/L to 355. Patients' 4 and 5 increased from 76 and 49 to 86 and 100, respectively.

A biopsy showed no evidence of disease in Patient 1, but Patient 2 had developed focal segmental glomerulosclerosis (FSGS): a disease that inhibits the kidney's ability to filter waste.

Podocytes are cells that encase the capillaries of the glomerulus (nerve endings around the kidney). Patient 3, who already had FSGS, was found to have contracted this condition.

Mesangial IgA deposits indicate nephropathy. Patients 4 and 5 had significant levels. The patients were successfully treated with cortisone though their serum creatinine tests revealed higher values than before the jab.

LIVER INJURIES

In addition to kidneys, liver disease has been noted, post-jab. This, unfortunately, is normal for new medical products. Hepatotoxicity is toxic liver disease; also a form of hepatitis.

One study notes that, in general: "Drug-induced hepatotoxicity leads to nearly 10% of all cases of acute hepatitis and more than 50% cases of liver failure." (The study then goes on to trumpet the jab.)[146]

Given the high prevalence of new and quickly withdrawn drugs causing liver damage, it is important to examine the Pfizer and other injections.

As noted in our previous chapters, FOIA-released documents prove that the company was negligent in following up on patient health surveillance, including deaths, after injection.

Referring to all companies' COVID-related injectable products, Hoo and the team note: "These vaccines caused rare side effects *not known during clinical trials*" (emphasis added).[147]

COVID increases the risk of acute liver injury. But what about the jab? A recent summary in *Nature* tells us that there is no risk of acute liver injury after injection.[148] But the original study, which also denies causation, says that 828 people per 100,000 double-dosed with Pfizer-BioNTech within 56 days developed diagnosed acute liver injury.[149] But what about undiagnosed injury?

It is normal scientific practice to compare cohorts: an injection-damaged group to a non-damaged group, for example. Yet, multiple papers suggesting injury omit comparative data.

Roy and the team studied post-jab immune-mediated liver injury in 23 patients acquired from a large dataset, though we don't know compared to who or how many.

Lymphoplasmacytic infiltrate can be a kind of rare, slow-acting cancer. Roy et al. found that this was the most common immune-mediated liver injury in the jabbed patients. Hepatocytes constitute most of the liver's known mass. Interface hepatitis is the death of those cells at certain sites. The researchers also found that interface hepatitis was a common post-injection phenomenon.[150]

The Israeli health officials' leaked Zoom call provides invaluable insight into long-term side-effects that are of no interest to Pfizer.

Chapter 11
How Pfizer Uses Children

In 2022, I wrote to both Pfizer and to the US Food and Drug Administration (FDA) to ask for information about their use of children in COVID vaccine experiments.

I wanted to know how many kids had been injected, what was their socioeconomic background (i.e., were children from poorer households and thus more likely to be exploited), and what compensation their parents/guardians received (i.e., were some parents selling their babies to Pfizer for money?).

"We are denying your entire request," replied Juris Doctor, Sarah Kotler, Director of the FDA's Division of Freedom of Information.

DENIAL

The exemptions cited included: "Information about individuals in personnel, medical and similar files when disclosure would constitute a clearly unwarranted invasion of privacy."

But, hang on, my original freedom of information (FOI) request clearly said that the patients' and parents/guardians' names and personal details can be redacted/anonymised.

Another reason cited was: "Trade secret and confidential commercial information."

But COVID and the experimental product are public health emergencies. What right do they have to deny the public information about a product injected into the public?

Secondly, my FOI asked for zero information about the product or the internal operations of Pfizer. My questions concerned what compensation, if any, parents/guardians received.

Laws cited included the Code of Federal Regulations and the Federal Trade Secrets Act.

To my surprise, Pfizer employees were more helpful.

PFIZER'S PUBLIC DATA

Olivia Campanella, Pfizer's Medical Information Associate, provided me with a document, which does not appear to be available online, on which most of this chapter is based.

My letter to Pfizer was open, my request to the FDA was a FOI submission. This is because, in the US, public bodies (the FDA) are subject to FOI and corporations (Pfizer) are not.

The injectable Pfizer product, BNT162b2, goes under the brand name Comirnaty. Its international non-proprietary name (or generic) is nucleoside-modified tozinameran.

"Comirnaty has been authorised under a 'conditional approval' scheme," said the information sheet in the body of the email.

In response to my question, neither the information sheet nor the attached document gave specific numbers, but did admit: "Pfizer offers reasonable payment for the time and effort to participate in a study."

So, there it is: Pfizer pays parents to inject their kids. Unlike the attached document, a quick search showed that this information sheet is available online.[151]

"In addition, Pfizer may offer reasonable payment to parents, guardians, or caregivers of minor children or incapacitated study participants."

As we shall see, the data show a high level of adverse events in babies and children who, according to other data, did not even need to be injected.

> Nominal gifts for study participation are allowed as long as the item does not display Pfizer (or affiliate) branding. For example, in studies involving minor children, a small, age-appropriate gift or gift certificate may be provided to the child.

So, Pfizer rewards pain, distress, and potential long-term damage in infants, toddlers, and children with toys.

With regards my question on the status of the kids: "socioeconomic background is not listed as part of the inclusion/exclusion criteria for Phase 1/2/3 Trial."

So, poorer families are at risk of being exploited for financial gain.

C.D.C AND PFIZER: CONTRADICTORY POSITIONS

In the US, the product is recommended by the Centers for Disease Control and Prevention (CDC) for children aged 6 months to 5 years.[152]

But the document I was given not only shows that Pfizer itself did *not* recommend giving under-5s the product, the trial was still in Phase I when the CDC issued the recommendation.

The US was an outlier: in other countries the jab is not (at the time of writing) recommended for under-5s in most Western countries.

According to the document I received: In March 2021, the Pfizer trials enrolled an "estimated" 11.4k kids aged 6 months to 12 years in the US, Finland, Poland, and Spain for a two-dose trial. (They don't even know for sure how many children they enrolled?)

Unhealthy children (whatever that's supposed to mean), were excluded from the study. But in the real world, children, like adults, suffer ill health. So, the efficacy of the product was artificially boosted because it was impossible to tell whether the product or the natural immunity of the children prevented COVID.

MIXING UP PHASES AND STAGES…AGAIN

Usually, Phase I includes pre-clinical trials, but as we've noted in other chapters, the company mixed up the trial phases.

For the kids, Phase I included five-to-12-year-old receiving 10 mcg doses and under-5s received 3 mcgs. Both age groups received a two-dose schedule.

With the document I was given last updated in July, the trial is still at Phase I.

In June 2022, the Vaccine and Related Biological Products Advisory Committee (US) met to discuss Emergency Use Authorization and approved the injection for 6 month to 5 year-olds.

According to the document, of the children who had two doses of the 10 mcgs (over 5s), 43.8 percent experienced adverse events.

Nearly one-in-five 5 to 11 year-olds experienced redness at the injection site.

For the 6 month to 23 month-old participants, 51.2 percent experienced post-injection irritability, 27 percent drowsiness, 22 percent decreased appetite, and 16 percent injection-site tenderness.

Of the 2 to 4 year-olds, one-in-three had pain at the injection site, a similar percentage had fatigue, and 11.4 percent redness.

In the 6 to 23 month cohort, three infants were withdrawn after experiencing pyrexia (severe fever). The document claims no heart-related adverse events were recorded, but then there appears to be a redaction in the form of an ellipsis in square brackets.

Despite the CDC pushing the product, Pfizer says:

> Post-licensure and post-authorization observational studies of Comirnaty and Pfizer-BioNTech COVID-19 Vaccine, respectively, have demonstrated decreased effectiveness of

a primary series against the currently predominant Omicron variant compared with effectiveness against the ancestral strain and variants (Alpha, Delta) that were predominant during pre-authorization trials in adults and older pediatric age groups.

SAFETY NOT YET ESTABLISHED

In June 2022, the CDC recommended the product under Emergency Use Authorization for under-5s.

Yet, the Pfizer document given to me was updated one month later in July.

It says: "The safety and efficacy of Comirnaty in paediatric children aged less than 5 years have not yet been established. Comirnaty is not approved for use in children aged less than 5 years."

Although that paragraph refers to February (before the CDC recommendation) it is important to stress that the document was updated in July. This created a discrepancy which no one seems to have noticed between Pfizer's own position and that of the CDC.

It is also important to reiterate that the CDC is an outlier because other governments--those of the EU and Australia, etc.--do not recommend the product to under-5s.

Rather appallingly, the CDC seems to have made its recommendation for under-5s to be jabbed on the basis of poor data given by Pfizer.

When it comes to a criterion called immunobridging, the Pfizer document I was given, referring to 6 month to four year-olds, says "some subgroups were too small to draw meaningful conclusions."

Another, Preliminary Descriptive Efficacy, notes that the type of infection was typically Omicron: the least severe to date.

Chapter 12
Pfizer Knew About Myocarditis

The January 2023 FDA/Pfizer releases contain some astonishing information confirming that the company marketed a dangerous experimental product, skipping Phase IV trials--which are usually long-term, large population safety studies--in favour of a speedy rollout under emergency use authorisation.

The documents confirm that the company knew about the increased risk of myocarditis but did not pull the product.[153]

Not only that, but the documents show track-changes in which both Pfizer and the US Food and Drug Administration (FDA) rewrote key words in the "Prescribing Information" sheet (for health professionals), the most serious of all adjustments appears to be the rounding down of adverse events to zero.

Documents also confirm that the company acknowledged that no trials had been undertaken to confirm the safety of mix-and-match injections and boosters--e.g., a Pfizer first schedule with an AstraZeneca booster. Yet, governments told us it was safe to combine different injectable products.

In development, the Pfizer-BioNTech injectable product was called BNT162b2. When it was marketed, the company named it Comirnaty.

DATA V PROPAGANDA

Documents include paperwork for the inserts as well as instructions for nurses. In theory, these were publicly-available documents, but the public never got to see them.

The "prescribing information" draft is dated August 2021, when medical professionals and propaganda were still denying a link between the injection and heart-related adverse events.

For instance, the *New York Times* ran with: "CDC is investigating heart problems in a few young COVID vaccine recipients."[154]

Notice the minimisation: "a few" and "young." A more accurate headline would be: "COVID injection increases risk of heart problems, particularly in young people."

But there was no need for public authorities to investigate. Rather, the product should have been pulled. Scandalously, the Pfizer papers were quite open. The prescribing information says:

> Postmarketing data demonstrate increased risks of myocarditis and pericarditis, particularly within 7 days following the second dose. The observed risk is higher among males under 40 years of age than among females and older males. The observed risk is highest in males 12 through 17 years of age. Although some cases required intensive care support, available data from short-term follow-up suggest that most individuals have

had resolution of symptoms with conservative management.[155]

Minus the "short-term" stipulation, the final sentence may sound somewhat reassuring, but consider the following line: "Information is not yet available about potential long-term sequelae" (a new condition triggered by previous injuries).

Another example of pro-injection propaganda circulating at the time, despite corporate internal warnings, is the *New York Times* stating: "Heart problems following vaccination in the U.S. are uncommon and short-lived, researchers reported."[156]

REPORT TO PFIZER FIRST

Appallingly, Pfizer advised medical professionals to report to the company in the first instance of patients experiencing adverse events. It recommended professionals contact the US government's Vaccine Adverse Event Reporting System (VAERS) second: "To report SUSPECTED ADVERSE REACTIONS, contact Pfizer Inc. at 1-800-438-1985 or VAERS at 1-800-822-7967 or http://vaers.hhs.gov."

Report to the company? Why? For damage control? Surely adverse events should, in the first instance, be reported to health authorities?

Recall American nurse, Tiffany Dover, who received a Pfizer injection live on air in order to promote the product, and then collapsed moments later?[157] Dover later claimed that she has a rare condition that causes her to faint when experiencing even mild pain.

But Pfizer's own prescribing information says: "Syncope (fainting) may occur in association with administration of injectable vaccines, including COMIRNATY. Procedures should be in place to avoid injury from fainting."

Quite amazingly and in a single paragraph, Pfizer debunks the entirety of its own clinical trials in relation to adverse events. The document says:

> Because clinical trials are conducted under widely varying conditions, adverse reaction rates observed in the clinical trials of a vaccine cannot be directly compared to rates in the clinical trials of another vaccine and may not reflect the rates observed in practice.

What? The real world is too complicated to accurately reflect the conditions of clinical trials? So, what was the point of the trials? This is why Phase IV studies usually exist: to apply laboratory conditions to everyday life.

Pfizer says that it did "not have a source table for non-serious AEs" (adverse events).

ROUNDING TO ZERO

Referring to a one-month period after the second dose for participants aged 16 to 55, the original line read: "In an analysis of serious and all adverse events..."

But Pfizer changed this to read: "In an analysis of all adverse events ..."

In other words, they minimised the wording to reduce reference to serious adverse events.

The percentages of Pfizer-to-placebo participants experiencing adverse events included 0.2 v. <0.01 who experienced decreased appetite, 0.1 v. <0.01 hyperhidrosis (excess sweating), 0.1 v. 0.01 lethargy, and night sweats 0.1 v. 0.01.

Pfizer rounded the placebo group to zero, so medical professionals therefore have no real way of comparing the rate of injection-related adverse events to the placebo group. In addition, it looks better on paper for Pfizer to have an adverse event ratio of 0.1 to 0 than 0.1 to 0.01 because the latter puts the former into context.

Interestingly, the FDA suggested "that the numbers in this paragraph [should] only include the non-serious adverse events." Perhaps wanting to protect their public image, Pfizer lobbied to keep the serious adverse event data in the particular paragraph.

Having exploded its own clinical trial data by saying that lab tests do not apply to the complexities of reality, Pfizer then writes:

The following adverse reactions have been identified during postmarketing use of

COMIRNATY, including under Emergency Use Authorization. Because these reactions are reported voluntarily from a population of uncertain size, it is not always possible to reliably estimate their frequency or establish a causal relationship to vaccine exposure.

Isn't that their job, along with the FDA and CDC?

They included: cardiac disorders, particularly myocarditis and pericarditis; gastrointestinal disorders (diarrhoea and vomiting); immune system disorders (angioedema, anaphylaxis, pruritus, rash, and urticaria (hives)); and musculoskeletal and connective tissue disorders.

PREGNANT

One final shocker: Pfizer did not bother to conduct long-term studies into the impact of the injection on pregnant women: "Available data on COMIRNARTY administered to pregnant women are insufficient to inform vaccine-associated risks in pregnancy."

But this not what the lying, fake news media told us. They consistently told naive, pregnant women that the injection was safe and necessary, even though the internal documents say that Pfizer and the FDA didn't even know.

In summary, Pfizer and/or the FDA:

- Rounded down patient data;

- Deleted passages in instructions to minimise reference to severe injury;

- Acknowledged that its trials had no real-world application in terms of measuring adverse events;

- Found adverse events post-marketing yet did not withdraw the product;

- Encouraged media and authorities to force pregnant women to get injected via "vaccine mandates" despite acknowledging that no safety data exist.

Chapter 13
Pfizer Downplayed Nanoparticle Dangers

Pfizer's partner, the German company BioNTech, published an internal 2,237-page report on its animal experiments. The report parses phrases, saying things like: there was no "systematic" lipid nanoparticle toxicity detected in the rodents. So, there *was* toxicity.[158]

In addition, the raw data are not included in the report. Their reference numbers are redacted and, under German law, will be kept secret for 15 years before being destroyed.

LIPID NANOPARTICLES

Lipids--or fats--naturally constitute cell membranes, regulate cell penetration, store vitamins, aid the production of hormones, and much more.[159]

A nanometre is one-billionth of a metre.[160] Nanoparticles can be organic, like volcanic dust, or human-made, such as carbon tubes. Their dimensions are between one and 100 nanometres.

Since the 1990s, scientists have experimented with modified lipid nanoparticles as a vehicle for novel therapeutics. The aim is to effectively hide the therapeutics in the lipids, like Trojan horses, so that the body does not reject the therapeutic. Once inside the cell, the therapeutic reproduces and in theory stimulates an immune response.

Messenger RNA (mRNA) mediates between genes and proteins. Antigens are molecules that bind to T-cells and antibodies, and typically trigger an immune response. The Pfizer-BioNTech injectable product is, in theory, an mRNA antigen.[161]

NEGATIVE CHARGES

Our bodies are electric. Negatively-charged cell surfaces are called anionic. mRNA membranes are anionic and thus rejected by cell membranes. The mRNA is thus encased in positively-charged lipid nanoparticles (cationic) that enter the given cell.[162]

As late as mid-2019, just prior to the pandemic, it was understood that "Lipid nanoparticles (LNPs) tend to accumulate in the liver." The study noting this important fact added: "the mechanisms that promote delivery to other cell types within the liver microenvironment are poorly understood."[163]

Yet, we are supposed to believe that Pfizer and BioNTech mastered this mystery within months to deliver a safe product.

The Pfizer-BioNTech product uses two types of lipids: PEGylated and phospholipids.[164]

PEG is polyethylene glycol. Pfizer, BioNTech, and governments allowed the experimental, genetically-modified mRNA lipid nanoparticle product to be injected into billions of people worldwide despite

PEG causing anaphylactic shock--a severe immune response--in people allergic to PEG.[165]

In addition to PEG, cationic lipids (positively-charged) were widely reported in the pre-COVID literature as being cytotoxic, i.e., toxic to cells, as we shall soon see.

But then governments declared a global pandemic and an apparently necessary rush to rollout an alleged vaccine based, in part, on cationic lipids, and suddenly the toxicity was forgotten.

Cationic (re)agents are abbreviated (+)NP, as in positively-charged nanoparticles. A study from 2010 said:

> Mice treated with (+)NPs showed increased liver enzyme release and body weight loss compared to mice treated with neutral or negatively charged NPs ((−)NPs), suggesting hepatotoxicity.[166]

The latter refers to liver toxicity.

NEGATIVELY-CHARGED PARTICLES AND TOXICITY

Eight years later, the safety of cationic agents was still in question. Lipids are non-viral vectors for gene therapy. A 2018 study--just a couple of years before the "vaccine" was rolled out--said: "As effective non-viral vectors …, cationic lipids still have the problem of toxicity, which has become one of the main bottlenecks for their applications."[167]

Another study from late-'19, just before the pandemic was announced, said: "cationic reagents are generally cytotoxic."[168]

The latest document dump contains thousands of pages downplaying the toxicity of lipid nanoparticles, apparently found in the organs of test animals.

The document was approved in September 2020.

BioNTech used 255 Han Wistar rats. Some were injected with failed vaccine candidates, others were injected with what became Comirnaty. Some were injected with a 30 µg dose, others with a 100.

So-called dose exposure is important because, in theory, vaccinologists aim to give the lowest dose with the highest efficacy.[169] But the BioNTech report says from the outset: "The analysis of dose exposure was conducted under the responsibility of the Sponsor is excluded from this statement."

So, how do we know what effect the dose exposure had?

THE SCIENCE WAS "FOGGY" THEN SUDDENLY SAFE

The first problem is that the report was rewritten at the request of the sponsor, but the report also claims that the rewrites did not make any substantive differences. This suggests a cover-up.

The second problem is that major mistakes were made in the first draft. This calls into question the accuracy of the second draft:

changes for albumin [protein made by the liver] and globulin [immune system-produced protein] levels were incorrectly stated as an increase in albumin and a decrease in globulin plasma levels instead of [vice versa].

Small activating RNAs are different from mRNAs, yet they interact in ways described as "foggy" just 18 months before the animal trials.[170]

The third problem is that the initial draft confused small activating RNAs with mRNAs. This is a serious problem if the tests were designed to study the effect of mRNA. Does this mean that the draft or the actual tests were confused?

The fourth problem was that the vaccine candidates ending in b1 and a1 were mixed up initial tables. Were the wrong candidates injected into the poor rats or merely reported incorrectly?

ADVERSE EVENTS IN ANIMALS

Despite being told that the injection was "safe and effective" for humans, the BioNTech report notes that many experimental rats had adverse reactions. But the language minimises the severity.

Depending on the dose number and potency, "a few" rats experienced "severe oedema" (swelling). Others endured erythema (skin inflammation). Some of the animals' skins had shed (eschar) to the point where the injection site had to be moved for the second and/or third doses.

Some rats suffered muscle death (necrosis) and fibrosis (tissue thickening or scarring).

In the females:

> Inflammation extended into tissues adjacent to the injection site, including mammary tissue, perineural [nerve group] tissue of sciatic nerve, tissue around the femur/knee and to the draining lymph node (iliac).

What appear to be mRNA and small activating RNA--we don't know which because the original draft was wrong--were present in the rodents:

> Test item-related microscopic findings at the end of dosing were evident in injection sites and surrounding tissues, increased cellularity of germinal centres [structures in white blood cells] and increased plasma cells in the draining (iliac) lymph nodes, bone marrow, spleen, and liver.

The report casually mentions "enlarged spleens."

BIODISTRIBUTION: UNKNOWN

People started getting mRNA injections from December 2020. But a study published as late as mid-2022 said: "The biodistribution and pharmacokinetics of the mRNA-containing lipid nanoparticles (LNPs) in these vaccines are unknown in humans."[171]

So, for nearly two years, billions of people had been injected, some multiple times, with a novel product whose distribution in their bodies was unknown. The study also said: "We found that vaccine-associated synthetic mRNA persists in systemic circulation for at least 2 weeks."

A recent article investigating myocarditis in adolescents and young people found elevated spike protein in their blood:

> markedly elevated levels of full-length spike protein ..., unbound by antibodies, were detected in the plasma of individuals with postvaccine myocarditis, whereas no free spike was detected in asymptomatic vaccinated control subjects.[172]

Another studied chronic hepatitis C virus (HCV) patients: "In 10 of 108 HCV patient samples, full-length or traces of SARS-CoV-2 spike mRNA vaccine sequences were found in blood up to 28 days after COVID-19 vaccination."[173]

Necrotising encephalitis (swelling) often results in brain lesions. Vasculitis describes blood vessel inflammation.

In October 2022, a study investigated the death of a Parkinson's Disease patient who had been injected three times. The first was with the non-mRNA Oxford-AstraZeneca jab, the second and third were with mRNA products. The patient had no history of having COVID-19.

> [H]istopathological analyses of the brain uncovered previously unsuspected findings, including acute vasculitis (predominantly lymphocytic) as well as multifocal necrotizing encephalitis of unknown etiology with pronounced inflammation including glial [central nervous system cells] and lymphocytic reaction.[174]

DECEPTIONS

Pre-COVID data on lipid nanoparticles (LNPs) suggested that they are toxic to cells and that reducing toxicity is not only difficult but has not been explored in clinical trials.

In addition, it was acknowledged in peer-reviewed medical literature that the distribution of LNPs and mRNA spike protein in humans was not understood.

Despite this, governments approved Pfizer-BioNTech's injectable product. The animal trial data suggest that toxicity was downplayed in the published reports.

Even more appalling, the products injected into the animals and the results were mixed up in the first draft, bringing the integrity of the second into serious question. Dose analyses were not even counted.

This had the effect of bringing an experimental product to a captive market under emergency use authorisation, when, in non-pandemic times, such risky products would never have been approved.

Chapter 14
Nearly Every Page Redacted

The document dump of April 2023 is arguably the most crucial to date, and thus the most censored. It should provide the raw data on the concentrations of antibodies in human blood stimulated by the injectable product.

But it doesn't.

Readers will be alarmed to see hundreds and hundreds of blank pages, redacted mainly under section (b)(4) of the US Freedom of Information Act: the protection of trade secrets.

It would seem that Pfizer/the FDA are hiding under (b)(4) to conceal the results of the injection trials, as well as its laboratory safety protocols.

If we had access to these data, we could interpret how well or poorly the alleged vaccine performed, and compare its performance to natural immunity.

WHAT ARE THEY HIDING?

In April 2023, Pfizer released over 50 documents. Most of them come from the Pfizer Vaccine Research and Development laboratory in Pearl River, New York. They concern the particulars of how the company analysed the results of its vaccine candidate trials.

But almost every single page is redacted, which renders rather meaningless the US judge's order: that the documents enter the public domain.

So, what is the company hiding?

In August last year, Annaliesa Anderson became head of Pfizer's Vaccine Research and Development.[175] Her previous work included leading the team of scientists that delivered the antiviral oral medication, Paxlovid, to emergency use authorization.

No sooner had Dr. Anderson taken up her new position, *Nature* published a shocking, non-clinical piece of public relations for Pfizer, authored by Dr. Anderson (details below).

The article was published just one month after Pfizer announced its plan to invest $470 million in its Pearl River vaccine facility;[176] one of the many sites overseen by Anderson.

REDACTED DEFINITIONS

April's documents are dated from mid-2020 and concern analyses conducted by the company at one of the sites now overseen by Dr. Anderson, Pearl River.

Pearl River is located in Rockland County, New York, about half way between Philadelphia and Hartford, Connecticut, on the east coast.

Pfizer says that "Pearl River scientists are currently working to develop vaccines against other major infectious diseases."[177]

IgG is Immunoglobulin G, the most common human antibody. Assays are assessments. Pfizer measured post-injection human antibodies by comparing them to the number of receptor-binding domain (RBD) proteins in the virus. RBDs form part of SARS-CoV-2's spike that enable the virus to lock onto cells and infect them.

Pfizer assessed them using ThermoFisher Scientific's Luminex machine.

A July 2020 document contains a Glossary which includes definitions, like Ag (antigen), LNB (laboratory notebook), and so on. But the definition of "Batch" is completely redacted.[178]

A specialist site describes batch-testing as the method of conducting multiple tests in order to save money: "One of the main advantages of batch testing is that it reduces costs."[179]

It also notes that such testing methods can "deliver more reliable generic results than if a sample is tested individually."

In other words, if "Batch" refers to this method in the documents, then Pfizer likely cut corners by batch-testing and reported on generic instead of patient-specific results.

MORE REDACTIONS

The definition of "dilution plating"--a technique used to estimate the number of specific organisms in a sample--is also redacted. Is this also because Pfizer cut corners, risking potential sample contamination?

In one instance, an entire acronym and its definition are redacted.

Being a giant corporation partly responsible for people's health, one might assume that Pfizer would be transparent about its safety protocols.

However, a link to the company's Safety Data Sheets, which employees are meant to consult, is redacted. Why? More strikingly, a link to the Pearl River Environmental Health and Safety Laboratory Manual is redacted.

Specific equipment names are also redacted. Why redact those but not redact the Luminex product? Is it because the equipment used was below the optimum quality grade? These include washing stations, plate washers, platform shakers, and equipment unknown because it has also been entirely redacted.

Buffers maximise the adsorption (adhesion of particles) of antigens onto plates for analysis. The entire section "Buffers" is redacted, as is half of the section on Procedure.

Microspheres are used for assaying. Presumably to protect patents, Pfizer redacted the entire section on microspheres. The sections on robotic and manual preparations are redacted, as are the Reference Standards.

QCS is quality control serum. Perhaps most disturbing of all, a section entitled Unknown Specimen and QCS is entirely redacted. Were the assessed samples contaminated? If so, with what and did this affect the outcomes of the analyses?

In a final insult, two names of the five signatories are redacted under section (4)(6): the right to privacy. What right do public servants have to *professional* privacy when they are developing a potentially dangerous health product used by billions of people?

THE SPEED OF SCIENCE

In the pro-pharma, *Nature* PR article mentioned above, Dr. Anderson acknowledges that pre-pandemic vaccine development and marketing used to take between 10 and 15 years.

In 2020, Paul Dabbar, Under Secretary of State at the US Department of Energy, said that American companies would work at the "speed of science" to develop a vaccine.[180] Thomas Gatliff, of Gatliff Technologies, quipped: The speed of science is:

"The velocity at which money flows from government bank accounts into the accounts of pharmaceutical company accounts."[181]

Dabbar's language coincided with the US government's effort to develop a vaccine, entitled Operation Warp Speed.

Returning to the *Nature* article mentioned above: In the same vein, Dr. Anderson more recently described Pfizer's approach as "lightspeed."[182]

Anderson says that Pfizer could get the injectable product out so quickly because government and Pfizer cleared away unnecessary bureaucracies, obliged different teams to work simultaneously instead of linearly, and based research and technology on decades-worth of prior research.

This new approach, she says, will enable new injectable mRNA products to get into human bodies quicker than ever before: "[It] provides real-world lessons on how to help avoid a regression to pre-pandemic ways."

NEW TECHNOLOGIES BASED ON DUBIOUS DATA

But "pre-pandemic" ways meant safety first via exercising the precautionary principle: hence the pulling from market of so many prior, failed vaccines.

In her article, Anderson leaves out a few things:

As we've seen in this book, the Pfizer papers show that the company mixed up stages with phases, unblinded their trials, failed to follow up on participant health and mortality, statistically rounded injuries (in some cases to zero), and secretly planned for a third dose while telling the world that two shots were "safe and effective."

If this is the method by which the company will move at "lightspeed" to bring new products to market, it might be better to go back to the previous method.

Pfizer says: "We strive to set the standard for quality, safety and value in the discovery, development and manufacture of health care products."[183]

But the latest batch of censored Pfizer papers does not allow us to verify this claim.

This chapter mainly quotes from the July 2020 document because, of all the Pearl River papers, it is one of the *least* redacted. Many of the documents (particularly from February 2021) consist almost entirely of redacted pages.

I contacted Dr. Anderson to ask why she thought that the documents were so heavily censored. Neither she nor her colleagues replied.

Conclusion
Our mRNA Future

It may soon be impossible to escape mRNA.

In 2003, the Bill and Melinda Gates Foundation launched its Grand Challenges in Global Health (GCGH) initiative. Five years later, the GCGH awarded Professor Hiroyuki Matsuoka of Jichi Medical University in Japan a reported one million dollars to design a genetically-modified mosquito.

There is no further reporting on the project, but the GMO mosquito will secrete malaria vaccine into the host's skin. In other words, Gates envisages a future in which mosquito bites are vaccines.[184]

This research ignored basic principles, like consent and informed decision, and creates an ethical minefield for injury claims.

Without further research, it is difficult to tell how much mRNA product has infected non-injected individuals.

Luigi Warren is the CEO of Cellular Reprogramming Inc. and a colleague of Moderna co-founder, Derrick Rossi.

In May 2021, Warren's Twitter account was suspended after he wrote that, although the load is "miniscule" and does not "cause disease/malaise in others," injected individuals do shed mRNA spike protein.[185]

BAD PATHS TO SCIENCE

It is widely reported that mRNA will replace non-mRNA vaccines. This future is terrifying. First, the COVID mRNA products were injected into captive populations based on faulty clinical trial data.

Second, the mRNA products had, by vaccine standards, extremely high rates of adverse events.

Third, no long term-studies have been conducted on what health impacts mRNA products have on the human body.

Fourth, medical professionals have become used to lowering design, development, and distribution standards because of the pandemic and the speed with which mRNA products were released to the public.

Fifth, perhaps most disturbing of all, because the injection-injured were hidden from the public due to de facto media censorship, the public generally thinks that the injections ended the pandemic, were safe, and were a big success.

As a result, people are now more likely to accept high-risk, low-regulation experimental products.

Six, it is possible that many people who might develop long-term injuries that they do not realise are related to the purported vaccine will take more mRNA therapeutics thinking that the new products will cure or help their existing ailments.

WHO FUNDS W.H.O.?

We have seen how the World Health Organization has long been co-opted by industry and private investors, notably Bill Gates.

In April 2023, the WHO boasted of its efforts to create global hubs for the development of mRNA technologies.

Many of these are in poorer countries with lax health regulations, repressive governments, and widespread poverty, meaning that publics who will serve as experimental subjects will not have the education or financial means to seek informed consent or compensation in the event of injury.

The aim, according to a WHO press release, is to research how mRNA might be adapted to purportedly fighting HIV and tuberculosis.[186]

The main company partnering with the WHO was the South African vaccine producer, Biovac, which has produced its own product, AfriVac 2121.

The Gates-funded GAVI published an article promoting the application of artificial intelligence in the design of purported vaccines. What could possibly go wrong?

The piece explains that programmes are being designed to "marry" mRNA to novel designs that could be clinically trialled within weeks of new pandemics.

In previous chapters, we noted how the World Economic Forum created the Coalition for Epidemic Preparedness Innovations (CEPI).

GAVI notes that CEPI is funding German researchers at the Institute of Drug Discovery to apply software to vaccine designs for the Nipah and Lassa viruses.[187]

MRNA IS UNSTABLE?

Simultaneously, China's tech giant, Baidu, is working its own algorithms to trigger antibodies 128 times greater than existing vaccines.

Dropping a bombshell, EuroNews reports that mRNA products are unstable because they are single stranded and can degrade more easily than DNA. MRNA degradation was not tested in the clinical trials.[188]

Burying the lead, the article then goes on to reiterate that cold storage is a problem for vaccines. The Chinese researchers are developing products that do not require such low temperatures and might be constructed like DNA to increase stability.

The French giant, Sanofi, has licensed the Chinese AI, LinearDesign.

In August 2023, the US giant Moderna announced that, making a reported $1 billion investment, it would develop mRNA technologies with China through a secret Memorandum of Agreement. Health Technology Report notes that Moderna's "strategic move into the Chinese market signifies a broader vision beyond COVID-19."[189]

In Australia, the biotech giant CSL has partnered with an American firm, Arcuturus Therapeutics, to develop mRNA vaccines. Ethan Settembre, Vice President of Research at CSL's Vaccine Innovation Unit, says: "it may be easier to have multiple vaccine strains in a single vaccine because each would require a lower dose."[190]

What could go wrong?

CHANGING THE GUIDELINES

Associate Professor Xiaowei Weng is head of the Molecular Imaging and Theranostics laboratory at the Baker Heart and Diabetes Institute, Australia.

In mid-2023, the Australian Department of Health and Aged Care published a puff piece promoting Dr. Weng's research into the use of mRNA to stop inflammation in blood vessels caused by, among other things, alcohol, fat, and smoking: and, one might add, certain injectable products.[191]

Inflicting their experiments on helpless animals, Weng's researchers are targeting the CD39 protein for modification via mRNA nanoparticles.

The Australian taxpayer, through the National Health and Medical Research Council's Medical Research Future Fund are footing some of the bill.

Around the same time, the European Medicines Agency drafted a concept paper on mRNA technologies. Based on existing clinical trial data, which this book as exposed as largely fraudulent, the goal is create regulations to bring mRNA infectious disease products to market.

The classification of mRNA depends, in part, on what is being targeted and whether the proteins are stimulated chemically or biologically. Existing guidelines do not account for these specifics.[192]

MRNA is being touted as a solution for other medical interventions. *Forbes* reports that mRNA could aid blood stem-cell transplant preparations.[193]

The theory is that mRNA could replace chemo- and radiation-therapies, as well as blood diseases like sickle cell and thalassemia.

The apparent source of the problem is hematopoietic stem cells. If damaged or mutated cells could be replaced with healthy ones, using mRNA technology, the disease will, theoretically, be ameliorated.

CRIMES

The Pfizer-BioNTech crime against humanity was not developing a novel, experimental vaccine candidate at "warp speed" (or at "the speed of science"). Rather, it was pushing people to get injected without informed consent.

Nothing in this book says that informed adults should refuse the injection. Instead, the book calls for basic protocol: that each recipient should have been made clear of the possible consequences and been able to make a risk-benefit analysis.

But that didn't happen. Big pharma colluded with government to economically coerce billions of people into being injected, even though many millions did not wish to be.

Those who wanted the injection and ended up getting seriously injured may not have been so keen to be injected had they known about the potential risks.

Those who did not wish to be injected under any circumstances found themselves forced into getting jabbed via mandates which blatantly violated the Nuremberg Code (see Appendix).

The virus against which the purported vaccine was supposed to protect overwhelmingly killed and hospitalised elderly and immune-compromised people. Yet, individuals who did not require vaccination ended up getting injected.

Consequently, hundreds of thousands of people, likely millions, have ended up with life-changing injuries as a result of big pharma's callous drive for profit.

Because vaccination is championed as by far the best, and for many the only solution, to public health crises, almost nobody in mainstream science or journalism has been willing to speak out on behalf of those who died or sickened as a result of an experimental injection forced upon them.

Medical Glossary

Albumin. A protein made by the liver.

Anaphylaxis. A potentially life-threatening immune system overreaction.

Arrhythmia. Irregular heartbeat.

Blinding. The purposeful concealment of group allocations from those involved in clinical research.

BNT162b1. A failed vaccine candidate that encodes for trimerised SARS-CoV-2 receptor-binding domain.

BNT162b2. An injectable product containing tozinameran riltozinameran, mRNA molecules programmed to reproduced SARS-CoV-2 proteins in the human body.

Cerebral edema. Brain swelling.

Cerebrovascular. Blood flow to the brain.

Clinical trial. A long-term, four phase study of dose ranges and side effects of new drugs and treatments on volunteers. (WHO definition, early-2020).

Confidence interval. Used in statistics, the mean of the estimate includes the addition and subtraction of the estimated variation.

Creatine. A chemical that supplies energy to muscles.

Creatinine. A chemical waste product of creatine.

Cytochrome c oxidase. An enzyme found in cell mitochondria.

DNA (Deoxyribonucleic acid). Polynucleotide chains that form a double helix, carrying genetic instructions enabling organisms to develop and function.

Enzymes. Proteins or RNA that convert molecules.

Erythema. Skin inflammation.

Fibroblasts. Cells that contribute to the connection of tissues.

Fibrosis. Tissue scarring or thickening.

Focal segmental glomerulosclerosis. A disease that inhibits the kidney's ability to filter waste.

Globulin. Immune system-produced protein.

Glomerulus. Nerve endings around the kidney.

Hepatotoxicity. Toxic liver disease.

Hypoesthesia. Numbness.

Immunity. The ability to resist specific disease by preventing the development of pathogenic organisms. (Pre-COVID definition, *Merriam-Webster's Medical Dictionary*, 1995 edition.)

In vitro. Tests performed in non-natural conditions, such as in test-tubes.

Ischaemic heart disease. Narrowing heart arteries that supply blood to the heart.

Lipids. Fatty compounds that include acids, glycerides, non-glycerides, and complex lipids.

Lymph nodes. Located in several parts of the body, they contain immune cells that attack infection.

Lymphadenopathy. Lymph node swelling.

Monomer. Molecules bond to others to form polymers.

mRNA (Messenger RNA). Single-stranded RNA that carries protein information from DNA in cell nuclei to cytoplasm where the codes are translated into amino acids.

Myocardial infarction (heart attack). Decreased or complete cessation of blood flow to the myocardium.

Myocarditis. Inflammation of the myocardium.

Myocardium. The heart's muscle layer found in the walls of the heart chambers, consisting of cardiomyocytes (cells responsible for heart contractions).

Nephropathy. Kidney deterioration.

Oedema. Swelling.

Paraesthesia. Localised paralysis.

PCR (polymerase chain reaction). A test that makes copies of (amplifies) a DNA sample so that analysts that identify it.

Pericarditis. Inflammation of the pericardium.

Pericardium. Tissue surrounding the heart.

Pharmacokinetics. How the body interacts with drugs.

Placebo. A substance with no apparent therapeutic effect used as a control to test new products.

Podocytes. Cells that encase the capillaries of the glomerulus.

Polymer. Chemical compounds comprised of molecules consisting of molecules of the same kind.

Precursor. A substance from which another is formed.

Prostaglandins. Lipids that aid blood flow, anti-inflammation, and contribute to tissue healing.

Pulmonary arteries. Vessels that send blood to the lungs.

Pulmonary embolism. Blockage of the pulmonary arteries.

RNA (Ribonucleic acid). Single-stranded nucleotides that assist the construction of cells, responding to immune challenges, and transporting amino acids intracellularly.

SARS-CoV-2. Severe acute respiratory syndrome coronavirus 2.

Severe adverse event (a.k.a., serious adverse reaction). A response to a medical product resulting in death, life-threatening injury, and/or persistent disability or incapacity, including birth defects. (European Medicines Agency.)

Tachycardia. A stress-related heart rate over 100 beats per minute, including the life-threatening supraventricular and ventricular tachycardia.

Thrombosis. Blood vessels blocked by clots. Venous thrombosis describe blood clots in veins and arterial describes clots in artery.

Trimer. A polymer consisting of three monomer units.

Trimerization. Chemical reactions that involve three identical molecules producing single trimers.

Unblinding. When staff and participants become aware of treatments and interventions assigned to trial participants.

Vaccine. A product that produces immunity to disease by stimulating the formation of specific antibodies. (Pre-COVID definition, Oxford Concise Medical Dictionary, 2015 edition.)

Vasculitis. Blood vessel inflammation.

Appendix

The Nuremberg Code (1949)

1. The voluntary consent of the human subject is absolutely essential. This means that the person involved should have legal capacity to give consent; should be so situated as to be able to exercise free power of choice, without the intervention of any element of force, fraud, deceit, duress, over-reaching, or other ulterior form of constraint or coercion; and should have sufficient knowledge and comprehension of the elements of the subject matter involved, as to enable him to make an understanding and enlightened decision. This latter element requires that, before the acceptance of an affirmative decision by the experimental subject, there should be made known to him the nature, duration, and purpose of the experiment; the method and means by which it is to be conducted; all inconveniences and hazards reasonably to be expected; and the effects upon his health or person, which may possibly come from his participation in the experiment. The duty and responsibility for ascertaining the quality of the consent rests upon each individual who initiates, directs or engages in the experiment. It is a personal duty and responsibility which may not be delegated to another with impunity.

2. The experiment should be such as to yield fruitful results for the good of society, unprocurable by other

methods or means of study, and not random and unnecessary in nature.

3. The experiment should be so designed and based on the results of animal experimentation and a knowledge of the natural history of the disease or other problem under study, that the anticipated results will justify the performance of the experiment.

4. The experiment should be so conducted as to avoid all unnecessary physical and mental suffering and injury.

5. No experiment should be conducted, where there is an a priori reason to believe that death or disabling injury will occur; except, perhaps, in those experiments where the experimental physicians also serve as subjects.

6. The degree of risk to be taken should never exceed that determined by the humanitarian importance of the problem to be solved by the experiment.

7. Proper preparations should be made and adequate facilities provided to protect the experimental subject against even remote possibilities of injury, disability, or death.

8. The experiment should be conducted only by scientifically qualified persons. The highest degree of skill and care should be required through all stages of the experiment of those who conduct or engage in the experiment.

9. During the course of the experiment, the human subject should be at liberty to bring the experiment to an end, if he has reached the physical or mental state, where continuation of the experiment seemed to him to be impossible.

10. During the course of the experiment, the scientist in charge must be prepared to terminate the experiment at any stage, if he has probable cause to believe, in the exercise of the good faith, superior skill and careful judgement required of him, that a continuation of the experiment is likely to result in injury, disability, or death to the experimental subject.

Endnotes

[1] Ehline Law Firm, "Government Pressure or Negligence?," no date, https://ehlinelaw.com/blog/pfizer-trial-hid-injuries.

[2] Emails to CCHVRC, https://downloads.regulations.gov/FDA-2021-N-1088-129763/attachment_2.pdf.

[3] Stephanie and Patrick de Garay, Docket No. FDA-2021-N-1088 for "Vaccines and Related Biological Products; Notice of Meeting," https://downloads.regulations.gov/FDA-2021-N-1088-129763/attachment_1.pdf.

[4] Jenna Greene, "Wait what? FDA wants 55 years to process FOIA request over vaccine data," Reuters, 18 November 2021, https://www.reuters.com/legal/government/wait-what-fda-wants-55-years-process-foia-request-over-vaccine-data-2021-11-18/.

[5] Deichmann et al. write of pre-COVID criteria: "The risks to human subjects unexpectedly outweigh the benefits because of unexpected severe adverse events. When the institutional review board (IRB) approves a trial, it has determined that it meets US Food and Drug Administration (FDA) criteria for IRB approval at 21 CFR 56.111. Section (a)(2) states: 'Risks to subjects are reasonable in relation to anticipated benefits, if any, to subjects, and the importance of the knowledge that may reasonably be expected to result.' This determination changes when a study unexpectedly causes serious illness or death in human subjects. The study may then be suspended by the

FDA, the sponsor, and/or the IRB until the risk-benefit ratio is reevaluated." Richard E. Deichmann, Marie Krousel-Wood and Joseph Breault (2016) "Bioethics in Practice: Considerations for Stopping a Clinical Trial Early," *The Ochsner Journal*, 16(3): 197–198.

[6] John-Paul Ford Rojas, "Pfizer sees revenues double to $81bn thanks to COVID-19 vaccine," Sky News, 8 February 2022, https://news.sky.com/story/pfizer-sees-revenues-double-to-81bn-thanks-to-covid-19-vaccine-12536328.

[7] Josh Holder, "Tracking Coronavirus Vaccinations Around the World," *New York Times*, 13 March 2023, https://www.nytimes.com/interactive/2021/world/covid-vaccinations-tracker.html.

[8] Our World in Data, "Coronavirus (COVID-19) Vaccinations," live document, https://ourworldindata.org/covid-vaccinations.

[9] Reliefweb, "Pfizer, BioNTech and Moderna making $1,000 profit every second while world's poorest countries remain largely unvaccinated," 16 November 2021, https://reliefweb.int/report/world/pfizer-biontech-and-moderna-making-1000-profit-every-second-while-world-s-poorest.

[10] Eric Sagonowsky, "Pfizer eyes higher prices for COVID-19 vaccine after the pandemic wanes: exec, analyst," *Fierce Pharma*, 23 February 2021, https://www.fiercepharma.com/pharma/pfizer-eyes-higher-covid-19-vaccine-prices-after-pandemic-exec-analyst.

[11] WHO COVID-19 Ethics and Governance Working Group, "COVID-19 and mandatory vaccination:

Ethical considerations," 30 May 2022, https://apps.who.int/iris/rest/bitstreams/1425927/retrieve.

[12] Matthew J. Belvedere, "Bill Gates: My 'best investment' turned $10 billion into $200 billion worth of economic benefit," 23 January 2019, https://www.cnbc.com/2019/01/23/bill-gates-turns-10-billion-into-200-billion-worth-of-economic-benefit.html.

[13] WHO, "How WHO is funded," https://www.who.int/about/funding.

[14] Erin Banco, Ashleigh Furlong and Lennart Pfahler, "How Bill Gates and partners used their clout to control the global Covid response — with little oversight," *Politico*, 14 September 2022, https://www.politico.com/news/2022/09/14/global-covid-pandemic-response-bill-gates-partners-00053969.

[15] Ibid.

[16] AAHRPP, "Building Trust One Shot at a Time," Fall 2021, http://www.aahrpp.org/education-news-and-events/advance-newsletter/fall-2021/first-article.

[17] Ibid.

[18] Ibid.

[19] Berkeley Lovelace, "Scientists worry whether Russia's 'Sputnik V' coronavirus vaccine is safe and effective," CNBC, 11 August 2020, https://www.cnbc.com/2020/08/11/scientists-worry-whether-russias-sputnik-v-coronavirus-vaccine-is-safe-and-effective.html.

[20] Frank Jordans, "Major European nations suspend use of AstraZeneca vaccine," Associated Press, 15 March 2021, https://apnews.com/article/germany-suspends-astrazeneca-vaccine-blood-clotting-0ab2c4fe13370c96c873e896387eb92f.

[21] Angus Liu, "AstraZeneca withdraws US COVID vaccine application, shifts focus to antibody treatments," *Fierce Pharma*, 10 November 2022, https://www.fiercepharma.com/pharma/astrazeneca-withdraws-us-covid-vaccine-application-focus-shifts-antibody-treatments.

[22] Joseph Ax, "Democrat Biden warns against rushing out coronavirus vaccine, says Trump cannot be trusted," Reuters, 16 September 2020, https://www.reuters.com/article/us-usa-election-biden-idUSKBN2671NW.

[23] Jen Christensen, "Past vaccine disasters show why rushing a coronavirus vaccine now would be 'colossally stupid'," CNN, 1 September 2020, https://edition.cnn.com/2020/09/01/health/eua-coronavirus-vaccine-history/index.html.

[24] Suzanna Smalley, "Doctors alarmed as FDA floats 'emergency use' of COVID-19 vaccine, bypassing trials," Yahoo! News, 1 September 2020, https://news.yahoo.com/doctors-alarmed-as-fda-floats-emergency-use-of-covid-vaccine-bypassing-trials-153153624.html.

[25] Paul D. Thacker (2021) "Covid-19: Researcher blows the whistle on data integrity issues in Pfizer's vaccine trial," BMJ, 375: doi.org/10.1136/bmj.n2635.

[26] Ibid.

[27] Ibid.

[28] Ibid.

[29] Ibid.

[30] *USA (Brook Jackson) v Ventavia* et al., Case 1:21-cv-00008-MJT Document 2 Filed 01/08/21, https://www.iambrookjackson.com/_files/ugd/9df0bc_7355a5ae426e4494adba8bcf7c864d15.pdf.

[31] Ibid.

[32] Ibid.

[33] Ibid.

[34] https://whatismyipaddress.com/ip/67.225.169.61.

[35] Data cited in Carl Zimmer, "2 Companies Say Their Vaccines Are 95% Effective. What Does That Mean?," *New York Times*, 20 November 2020, https://web.archive.org/web/20201120170425/https://www.nytimes.com/2020/11/20/health/covid-vaccine-95-effective.html and Sarah Boseley, "Pfizer Covid-19 vaccine has 95% efficacy and is safe, further analysis shows," *Guardian*, 18 November 2020, https://www.theguardian.com/world/2020/nov/18/pfizer-covid-19-vaccine-95-effective-and-safe-further-tests-show.

[36] Katie Thomas, *NYT*, 18 November 2020, https://web.archive.org/web/20201231082321/https://www.nytimes.com/2020/11/18/health/pfizer-covid-vaccine.html.

[37] Erika Edwards, "FDA: Pfizer's Covid-19 vaccine safe and effective after one dose," NBC, 8 December 2020, https://www.nbcnews.com/health/health-news/fda-pfizer-s-covid-19-vaccine-safe-effective-after-one-n1250337.

[38] https://www.fda.gov/media/144245/download.

[39] Fernando P. Polack et al. (2020) "Safety and Efficacy of the BNT162b2 mRNA Covid-19 Vaccine," *New England Journal of Medicine*, 383: 2603-2615. Tragi-comically, it says: "Dr. Bennett, being employed by and owning stock and stock options in Moderna; Dr. Pajon, being employed by and owning stock in Moderna; Dr. Knightly, being employed by and owning stock and stock options in Moderna; Drs. Leav, Deng, and Zhou being employees of Moderna; Dr. Han, being employed by and owning stock and stock options in Moderna; Dr. Ivarsson, being employed by and owning share options in Moderna; Dr. Miller, being employed by and owning stock and stock options in Moderna; and Dr. Zaks, being employed by and owning stock options in Moderna. No other potential conflict of interest relevant to this article was reported."

[40] Peter Doshi, "Pfizer and Moderna's '95% effective' vaccines—we need more details and the raw data," BMJ Opinion, 4 January 2021, https://blogs.bmj.com/bmj/2021/01/04/peter-doshi-pfizer-and-modernas-95-effective-vaccines-we-need-more-details-and-the-raw-data/.

[41] Lindsey R. Baden et al. (2021) "Efficacy and Safety of the mRNA-1273 SARS-CoV-2 Vaccine," *New England Journal of Medicine*, 384(5): 403-16.

[42] Doshi, op. cit.

[43] Doshi, op. cit.

[44] Doshi, op. cit.

[45] Doshi, op. cit.

[46] Pfizer, "Vaccine information sheet," https://phmpt.org/wp-

content/uploads/2023/08/125742_S144_M1_lab-1451-11-0.pdf.

[47] Brighton Collaboration, "History," no date, https://brightoncollaboration.us/history/.

[48] CEPI, "Our Mission," no date, https://cepi.net/about/whyweexist/.

[49] Joseph Fraiman et al. (2022) "Serious adverse events of special interest following mRNA COVID-19 vaccination in randomized trials in adults," *Vaccine*, 40(40): 5798–5805.

[50] Ibid.

[51] Ioannis P. Trougakos et al. (2022) "Adverse effects of COVID-19 mRNA vaccines: the spike hypothesis," *Trends in Molecular Medicine*, 28(7): 542-554.

[52] Ming-Ming Yan et al. (2022) "Serious adverse reaction associated with the COVID-19 vaccines of BNT162b2, Ad26.COV2.S, and mRNA-1273: Gaining insight through the VAERS," *Frontiers in Pharmacology*, 13: 921760.

[53] Pratibha Anand and Vincent P. Stahel (2021) "Review the safety of Covid-19 mRNA vaccines: a review," *Patient Safety in Surgery*, 15: 20.

[54] Miguel García-Grimshaw et al. (2021) "Neurologic adverse events among 704,003 first-dose recipients of the BNT162b2 mRNA COVID-19 vaccine in Mexico: A nationwide descriptive study," *Clinical Immunology*, 229: 108786.

[55] Freise et al. (2022) "Acute cardiac side effects after COVID-19 mRNA vaccination: a case series," *European Journal of Medical Research*, 27(1): 80.

[56] Noam Barda et al. (2021) "Safety of the BNT162b2 mRNA Covid-19 Vaccine in a Nationwide Setting,"

New England Journal of Medicine, 385(12): 1078-1090.

[57] Carlos King Ho Wong et al. (2022) "Adverse events of special interest and mortality following vaccination with mRNA (BNT162b2) and inactivated (CoronaVac) SARS-CoV-2 vaccines in Hong Kong: A retrospective study," *PLoS Medicine*, 19(6): e1004018.

[58] Nicola P. Klein et al. (2021) "Surveillance for Adverse Events After COVID-19 mRNA Vaccination," *Journal of the American Medical Association*, 326(14): 1–10.

[59] Farah Yasmin et al. (2023) "Adverse events following COVID-19 mRNA vaccines: A systematic review of cardiovascular complication, thrombosis, and thrombocytopenia," *Immunity, Inflammation and Disease*, 11(3):e807.

[60] Casey B. Mulligan et al. (2022) "The Young were not Spared: What Death Certificates Reveal about Non-Covid Excess Deaths," *Inquiry*, 59: doi/epub/10.1177/00469580221139016.

[61] Barry Buzan and Gautam Sen (1990) "The Impact of Military Research and Development Priorities on the Evolution of the Civil Economy in Capitalist States," *Review of International Studies*, 16(4): 321-39.

[62] Department of Defense, "New Biotechnology Executive Order Will Advance DoD Biotechnology Initiatives for America's Economic and National Security," 14 September 2022, https://www.defense.gov/News/Releases/Release/Arti

cle/3157504/new-biotechnology-executive-order-will-advance-dod-biotechnology-initiatives-fo/.

[63] A. Liljas et al. (2022) "Messenger RNA (mRNA) based delivery into T cells provides a transient expression of the CAR gene," *Methods in Cell Biology*: https://www.sciencedirect.com/topics/medicine-and-dentistry/messenger-rna.

[64] Evanthia Tourkochristou (2021) "The Influence of Nutritional Factors on Immunological Outcomes," *Frontiers in Immunology*, 12: doi.org/10.3389/fimmu.2021.665968.

[65] Elie Dolgin, "The tangled history of mRNA vaccines," *Nature*, 14 September 2021, https://web.archive.org/web/20210918113900/https://www.nature.com/articles/d41586-021-02483-w.

[66] James K. Choung, "Regulation of COLx1(1), LO and COX-1 mRNA Expression by Prostaglandin E2 in Human Embryonic Fibroblasts, IMR-90," 1 January 1998, ADA349483, https://apps.dtic.mil/sti/pdfs/ADA349483.pdf.

[67] Steve F. Abcouwer, "Demonstration that a mRNA Binding Protein is Responsible for GADD45 mRNA Destabilization," University of New Mexico Health Sciences Center, U.S. Army Medical Research and Materiel Command Fort Detrick, Maryland, https://apps.dtic.mil/sti/pdfs/ADA418512.pdf.

[68] DARPA, "Driving Technological Surprise: DARPA's Mission in a Changing World," April 2013, https://defenseinnovationmarketplace.dtic.mil/wp-content/uploads/2018/02/DARPAStrategicPlan.pdf.

[69] Mohit Kumar (2018) "Amino-acid-encoded biocatalytic self-assembly enables the formation of transient conducting nanostructures," *Nature Chemistry*, 10: 696-703.

[70] Department of Defense, *Fiscal Year (FY) 2013 President's Budget Submission, Defense Advanced Research Projects Agency Justification Book Volume 1*, https://www.darpa.mil/attachments/(2G4)%20Global%20Nav%20-%20About%20Us%20-%20Budget%20-%20Budget%20Entries%20-%20FY2013%20(Approved).pdf.

[71] DARPA, *Young Faculty Awardees: Class of 2016*, https://www.darpa.mil/attachments/YFAClassof2016.pdf.

[72] Shannon Greene, "PReemptive Expression of Protective Alleles and Response Elements (PREPARE)," DARPA, no date, https://www.darpa.mil/program/preemptive-expression-of-protective-alleles-and-response-elements.

[73] Kathryn A. Whitehead, CV, http://whitehead.cheme.cmu.edu/ewExternalFiles/Whitehead%20CV%20-%20August%202022.pdf.

[74] Filippa Lentzos and Jez Littlewood, "DARPA's Prepare program: Preparing for what?," *Bulletin of the Atomic Scientists*, 26 July 2018, https://thebulletin.org/2018/07/darpas-prepare-program-preparing-for-what/.

[75] Alexander Bukreyev, "Development of a Modified mRNA-Based Vaccine for Lassa Virus," U.S. Army Medical Research and Development Command Fort

Detrick, Maryland, October 2020,
https://apps.dtic.mil/sti/pdfs/AD1116972.pdf.

[76] DARPA, "A Dose of Inner Strength to Survive and Recover from Potentially Lethal Health Threats," 27 June 2019, https://www.darpa.mil/news-events/2019-06-27.

[77] DARPA, "Preventing Pandemics," 29 January 2021, https://www.darpa.mil/attachments/Preventing_Pandemics_Vignette_Final_210208.pdf.

[78] Office of Public Relations, "Justice Department Announces Largest Health Care Fraud Settlement in Its History," Department of Justice (US), 2 September 2009, https://www.justice.gov/opa/pr/justice-department-announces-largest-health-care-fraud-settlement-its-history.

[79] Ibid.

[80] Ibid.

[81] Ibid.

[82] Good Jobs First, "Violation Tracker Current Parent Company Summary," Violation Tracker, no date, https://violationtracker.goodjobsfirst.org/parent/pfizer.

[83] CDC Foundation, Donors, Fiscal Year 2020, https://www.cdcfoundation.org/FY2020/donors.

[84] *Yahoo Finance*, "2 FDA officials reportedly resign over Biden administration booster-shot plan," 1 September 2021, https://finance.yahoo.com/video/vaccine-leaders-resign-pfizer-booster-142824241.html.

[85] *Washington Post Live*, "Albert Bourla on why mRNA technology was 'counterintuitive' to

producing an effective vaccine," 10 March 2022, https://www.youtube.com/watch?v=t9_YRw7jBF4.
[86] Cheyenne Haslett, "Fauci says COVID-19 cases will likely increase soon, though not necessarily hospitalizations," ABC News, 18 March 2022, https://abcnews.go.com/Politics/fauci-covid-19-cases-increase-necessarily-hospitalizations/story?id=83509114.
[87] United States District Court Northern District of Texas, PHTMPT v FDA, Case 4:21-cv-01058-P Document 1 Filed 09/16/21, https://phmpt.org/wp-content/uploads/2021/11/091621-Complaint.pdf.
[88] United States District Court Northern District of Texas, PHTMPT v FDA, Case 4:21-cv-01058-P Document 20 Filed 11/15/21, https://web.archive.org/web/20211123172128/https:/fingfx.thomsonreuters.com/gfx/legaldocs/egvbkaeggpq/vaccine%20foia%20status%20report.pdf.
[89] United States District Court Northern District of Texas, PHTMPT v FDA, United States District Court Northern District of Texas, PHTMPT v FDA, https://web.archive.org/web/20220110060733/https:/fingfx.thomsonreuters.com/gfx/legaldocs/gdvzykdllpw/Pittman%20FOIA%20Order.pdf.
[90] For example: Pfizer Worldwide Safety, "5.3.6. Cumulative analysis of post-authorization adverse event reports of PF-07302048 (BNT162B2) received through 28-Feb-2021," FDA-CBER-2021-5683-0000054, https://phmpt.org/wp-content/uploads/2021/11/5.3.6-postmarketing-experience.pdf.
[91] Merriam-Webster, "Definition of vaccine," online edition, 23 January 2017,

https://web.archive.org/web/20170123225217/https:/
www.merriam-webster.com/dictionary/vaccine.

[92] Merriam-Webster, "Vaccine," online edition, live document, https://www.merriam-webster.com/dictionary/vaccine.

[93] BNT162b2, "2.4 Nonclinical Overview," 8 February 2021, FDA-CBER-2021-5683-0013861, https://phmpt.org/wp-content/uploads/2022/03/125742_S1_M2_24_nonclinical-overview.pdf.

[94] Josh Holder, "Tracking Coronavirus Vaccinations Around the World," *New York Times*, 13 March 2023, https://web.archive.org/web/20230630120123/https://www.nytimes.com/interactive/2021/world/covid-vaccinations-tracker.html.

[95] Matej Mikulic, "Number of COVID-19 vaccine doses administered in the United States as of April 26, 2023, by vaccine manufacturer," Statista, 2 May 2023, https://www.statista.com/statistics/1198516/covid-19-vaccinations-administered-us-by-company/.

[96] *Clinical Study Data Reviewer's Guide BLA Analysis for Participants ≥16 Years of Age BioNTech SE and PFIZER INC.*, Study C4591001, 29 April 2021, https://phmpt.org/wp-content/uploads/2022/05/125742_S1_M5_c4591001-S-csdrg.pdf.

[97] Eleanor M Dinnett et al. (2005) "Unblinding of trial participants to their treatment allocation: lessons from the Prospective Study of Pravastatin in the Elderly at Risk (PROSPER)," *Clinical Trials*, 3:254-9.

[98] International Federation of Pharmaceutical Manufacturers and Associations (2019) *The Complex Journey of a Vaccine: The Steps Behind Developing a New Vaccine*, https://web.archive.org/web/20200501110007/https://www.ifpma.org/wp-content/uploads/2019/07/IFPMA-ComplexJourney-2019_FINAL.pdf.

[99] Pfizer, "Pfizer and BioNTech Dose First Participants in the U.S. as Part of Global COVID-19 mRNA Vaccine Development Program," 5 May 2020, https://web.archive.org/web/20200501110007/https://www.ifpma.org/wp-content/uploads/2019/07/IFPMA-ComplexJourney-2019_FINAL.pdf.

[100] Edward L. Korn and Boris Freidlin (2011) "Outcome-Adaptive Randomization: Is It Useful?," *Journal of Clinical Oncology*, 29(6): 771-76.

[101] Jacqueline French et al. (2014) "Pregabalin monotherapy in patients with partial-onset seizures," *Neurology*, 82: 590-97.

[102] Spencer Phillips Hey and Jonathan Kimmelman (2016) "Are Outcome-Adaptive Allocation Trials Ethical?," *Clinical Trials*, 12(2): 102-06.

[103] Ibid.

[104] Ibid.

[105] BNT162b2, "2.5 Clinical Overview," 30 April 2021, FDA-CBER-2021-5683-0002381, https://phmpt.org/wp-content/uploads/2022/06/STN-125742-0-0-Section-2.5-Clinical-Overview-reissue.pdf.

[106] Ibid.

[107] World Economic Forum, "Preparing for the Next Pandemic with Bill Gates," 24 May 2022, https://www.youtube.com/watch?v=NA0Fphx4UMg.

[108] Yahoo Finance, "Pfizer CEO: New COVID-19 vaccine that covers Omicron 'will be ready in March'," 10 January 2022, https://www.youtube.com/watch?v=lhMbKyDq9_w.

[109] Pfizer, "Pfizer and BioNTech Confirm High Efficacy and No Serious Safety Concerns Through Up to Six Months Following Second Dose in Updated Topline Analysis of Landmark COVID-19 Vaccine Study," 1 April 2021, https://www.pfizer.com/news/press-release/press-release-detail/pfizer-and-biontech-confirm-high-efficacy-and-no-serious.

[110] Berkeley Lovelace, "Pfizer CEO says third Covid vaccine dose likely needed within 12 months," CNCB, 15 April 2021, https://www.cnbc.com/2021/04/15/pfizer-ceo-says-third-covid-vaccine-dose-likely-needed-within-12-months.html.

[111] S.K. Agarwal (1999) "Comparison of two schedules of hepatitis B vaccination in patients with mild, moderate and severe renal failure," *Journal of the Association of Physicians of India*, 47(2):183-5.

[112] J. Taranger et al. (1999) "Vaccination of infants with a four-dose and a three-dose vaccination schedule," *Vaccine*, 18(9-10):884-91.

[113] Rajeev Zachariah Kompithra et al. (2014) "Immunogenicity of a three dose and five dose oral human rotavirus vaccine (RIX4414) schedule in south

Indian infants," *Vaccine*, 11(32): doi: 10.1016/j.vaccine.2014.03.002.

[114] Mark Jit et al. (2015) "Comparison of two dose and three dose human papillomavirus vaccine schedules: cost effectiveness analysis based on transmission model," BMJ, 350(7584): doi: 10.1136/bmj.g7584.

[115] Joon Young Song et al. (2020) "Immunogenicity and safety of a modified three-dose priming and booster schedule for the Hantaan virus vaccine (Hantavax): A multi-center phase III clinical trial in healthy adults," *Vaccine*, 38(50):8016-8023.

[116] Anu Kantele et al. (2022) "Three-dose versus four-dose primary schedules for tick-borne encephalitis (TBE) vaccine FSME-immun for those aged 50 years or older: A single-centre, open-label, randomized controlled trial," Vaccine, 40(9):1299-1305.

[117] Alasdair P.S. Munro et al. (2021) "Safety and immunogenicity of seven COVID-19 vaccines as a third dose (booster) following two doses of ChAdOx1 nCov-19 or BNT162b2 in the UK (COV-BOOST): a blinded, multicentre, randomised, controlled, phase 2 trial," *The Lancet*, 398(10318): doi.org/10.1016/S0140-6736(21)02717-3.

[118] https://pdata0916.s3.us-east-2.amazonaws.com/pdocs/070122/125742_S1_M5_5351_c4591001-interim-mth6-adverse-events.zip.

[119] Pfizer, "Compound: PF-07302048; Protocol: C4591001," FDA-CBER-2021-5683-0221179, 22 November 2020, https://pdata0916.s3.us-east-2.amazonaws.com/pdocs/070122/125742_S1_M5_5351_c4591001-fa-interim-narrative-sensitive.pdf.

[120] Pfizer Worldwide Safety, "5.3.6 Cumulative Analysis of Post-authorization Adverse Event Reports," FDA-CBER-2021-5683-0000054, 30 April 2021, https://phmpt.org/wp-content/uploads/2021/11/5.3.6-postmarketing-experience.pdf.

[121] Sharon H.X. Tan et al. (2022) "Effectiveness of BNT162b2 Vaccine against Omicron in Children 5 to 11 Years of Age," *New England Journal of Medicine*, 387: 525-32.

[122] Matthew E. Oster et al. (2022) "Myocarditis Cases Reported After mRNA-Based COVID-19 Vaccination in the US From December 2020 to August 2021," JAMA, 327(4):331-40.

[123] Elyse O. Kharbanda et al. (2021) "Spontaneous Abortion Following COVID-19 Vaccination During Pregnancy," JAMA, 326(16): 1629-31.

[124] Antonio Simone Laganà et al. (2022) "Evaluation of menstrual irregularities after COVID-19 vaccination: Results of the MECOVAC survey," *Open Medicine*, 17(1): 475–484.

[125] The letters are not now easy to find, including on Archive.org, but most of the text seems to be cut and paste into newer letters. See, for instance, FDA, Letter to Pfizer, 28 April 2023, https://www.fda.gov/media/150386/download.

[126] FDA Briefing Document, Pfizer-BioNTech COVID-19 Vaccine, *Vaccines and Related Biological Products Advisory Committee Meeting*, 10 December 2020, https://www.fda.gov/media/144245/download.

[127] Ibid.

[128] CDC, "Provisional COVID-19 Deaths by Sex and Age," 2 June 2022, https://web.archive.org/web/20220617111924/https://data.cdc.gov/NCHS/Provisional-COVID-19-Deaths-by-Sex-and-Age/9bhg-hcku.

[129] Pfizer, "Pfizer and BioNTech Initiate Rolling Submission for Emergency Use Authorization of Their COVID-19 Vaccine in Children 6 Months Through 4 Years of Age Following Request From U.S. FDA," 1 February 2022, https://www.pfizer.com/news/press-release/press-release-detail/pfizer-and-biontech-initiate-rolling-submission-emergency.

[130] Tan et al., op. cit.

[131] Jennifer Block, "Covid-19: US tracker overestimated deaths among children," BMJ, 376:831.

[132] Readers can put the key words and dates into *New York Times* Archive.

[133] A. Fabre and M.N. Sheppard (2006) "Sudden adult death syndrome and other non-ischaemic causes of sudden cardiac death," *BMJ*, 92(3): dx.doi.org/10.1136/hrt.2004.045518.

[134] ITV, "Cormac Trust supporting new research into sudden adult death syndrome at NUI Galway," 11 January 2022, https://www.itv.com/news/utv/2022-01-11/cormac-trust-supporting-new-research-into-sudden-adult-death-syndrome-in-galway.

[135] Office for National Statistics, "Sudden Adult Deaths 2016 to 2021," 22 December 2021, FOI/2021/3309,

https://www.ons.gov.uk/aboutus/transparencyandgov
ernance/freedomofinformationfoi/suddenadultdeaths2
016to2021.

[136] Lords, "Sudden Adult Death Syndrome," 9 June 2021, Vol. 812,
https://hansard.parliament.uk/Lords/2021-06-
09/debates/71DD9CA3-12BD-4EEF-98B8-
FDBFD1EA6B8D/SuddenAdultDeathSyndrome.

[137] Ibid.

[138] Will Feuer, "Pfizer's CEO hasn't gotten his Covid vaccine yet, saying he doesn't want to cut in line," CNBC, 14 December 2020,
https://www.cnbc.com/2020/12/14/pfizers-ceo-hasnt-
gotten-his-covid-vaccine-yet-saying-he-doesnt-want-
to-cut-in-line.html.

[139] Pfizer, "Statement from Pfizer Chairman and CEO Albert Bourla on Testing Positive for COVID-19," 15 August 2022,
https://www.pfizer.com/news/announcements/stateme
nt-pfizer-chairman-and-ceo-albert-bourla-testing-
positive-covid-19.

[140] Marek Glezerman, "Why Israel's Vaccine Deal With Pfizer Has Nothing to Do With Clinical Trials," *Haaretz*, 14 September 2021,
https://www.haaretz.com/opinion/2021-09-14/ty-
article-opinion/.premium/much-ado-about-israel-
pfizer-deal/0000017f-db80-df62-a9ff-dfd7bed30000.

[141] MOH-Pfizer Collaboration Agreement (Redacted), "Real-World Epidemiological Evidence Collaboration Agreement,"
https://web.archive.org/web/20210117134943/https:/g

ovextra.gov.il/media/30806/11221-moh-pfizer-collaboration-agreement-redacted.pdf.

[142] Daniel Estrin, "Vaccines For Data: Israel's Pfizer Deal Drives Quick Rollout — And Privacy Worries," NPR, 31 January 2021, https://www.npr.org/2021/01/31/960819083/vaccines-for-data-israels-pfizer-deal-drives-quick-rollout-and-privacy-worries.

[143] Available at "Israel Leak Number 4," https://www.bitchute.com/video/7rUpeAaI5Qwe/.

[144] Cited in Stuart McDonald, "Why have there been excess deaths this summer?," 24 August 2022, https://ukandeu.ac.uk/why-have-there-been-excess-deaths-this-summer/.

[145] Cecilia Czerlau et al. (2022) "Acute interstitial nephritis after messenger RNA-based vaccination," *Clinical Kidney Journal*, 15(1): 174-76.

[146] Rupinder Mann et al. (2021) "Drug-Induced Liver Injury After COVID-19 Vaccine," *Cureus*, 13(7): e16491.

[147] Chai-Zhen Hoo (2022) "Severe Hepatocellular Liver Injury After COVID-19 Vaccination Without Autoimmune Hepatitis Features: A Case Series," *ACG Case Reports Journal*, 9(4): e00760.

[148] Katrina Ray (2022) "No increased risk of acute liver injury after COVID-19 vaccination," *Nature Reviews Gastroenterology and Hepatology*, 19: 556.

[149] Carlos King Ho Wong et al. (2022) "Risk of acute liver injury following the mRNA (BNT162b2) and inactivated (CoronaVac) COVID-19 vaccines," *Journal of Hepatology*, 77(5): 1339-48.

[150] Akash Roy et al. (2022) "Immune-mediated liver injury following COVID-19 vaccination: A systematic review," *Hepatology Communications*, 6(9): 2513-22.

[151] Pfizer, "Payment and Reimbursement to Study Participants," no date, https://www.pfizer.com/science/clinical-trials/integrity-and-transparency/payment-reimbursement-participants.

[152] CDC, "CDC Recommends COVID-19 Vaccines for Young Children," 18 June 2022, https://www.cdc.gov/media/releases/2022/s0618-children-vaccine.html.

[153] Pfizer, "Vaccine Information Fact Sheet...," https://phmpt.org/wp-content/uploads/2023/08/125742_S144_M1_lab-1451-11-0.pdf.

[154] *New York Times*, "C.D.C. Is Investigating a Heart Problem in a Few Young Vaccine Recipients," 22 May 2021, https://www.nytimes.com/2021/05/22/health/cdc-heart-teens-vaccination.html.

[155] Pfizer, "Prescribing Information," August 2021, https://phmpt.org/wp-content/uploads/2023/01/125742_S70_M1_lab-1448-0-7-annotated.pdf.

[156] Apoorva Mandavilli, "Heart problems following vaccination in the U.S. are uncommon and short-lived, researchers reported," *New York Times*, 4 August 2021, https://web.archive.org/web/20210804211004/https://

www.nytimes.com/2021/08/04/health/myocarditis-covid-vaccine.html.

[157] Yaron Steinbuch, "Nurse faints while talking to press about getting COVID-19 vaccine," *New York Post*, 18 December 2020, https://nypost.com/2020/12/18/nurse-faints-while-talking-to-press-about-getting-covid-19-vaccine/.

[158] BioNTech, "Repeat-dose Toxicity Study...," Report No. 38166, Amendment No. 1, 1 July 2020, https://pdata0916.s3.us-east-2.amazonaws.com/pdocs/030123/125742_S1_M4_4.2.3.2+38166.pdf.

[159] J. Abraham Domínguez-Avila et al. (2020) "Lipids," *Progress in Molecular Biology and Translational Science*, https://www.sciencedirect.com/topics/agricultural-and-biological-sciences/lipids.

[160] National Nanotechnology Initiative, "Size of the Nanoscale," no date, https://www.nano.gov/nanotech-101/what/nano-size.

[161] Xucheng Hou et al. (2021) "Lipid nanoparticles for mRNA delivery," *Nature Reviews Materials*, 6: 1078-94.

[162] Editorial, "Let's talk about lipid nanoparticles," *Nature Reviews Materials*, 6: 99.

[163] Cory D. Sago et al. (2019) "Cell Subtypes Within the Liver Microenvironment Differentially Interact with Lipid Nanoparticles," *Celluar and Molecular Bioengineering*, 12(5): 389–397.

[164] Linde Schoenmaker et al., "mRNA-lipid nanoparticle COVID-19 vaccines: Structure and

stability," *International Journal of Pharmaceutics*, 601: 120586.

[165] Morgan D. McSweeney et al. (2021) "Anaphylaxis to Pfizer/BioNTech mRNA COVID-19 Vaccine in a Patient With Clinically Confirmed PEG Allergy," *Drug, Venom and Anaphylaxis*, 2: doi.org/10.3389/falgy.2021.715844.

[166] Ranit Kedmi et al. (2010) "The systemic toxicity of positively charged lipid nanoparticles and the role of Toll-like receptor 4 in immune activation," *Biomaterials*, 31(26): 6867-75.

[167] Shaohui Cui et al. (2018) "Correlation of the cytotoxic effects of cationic lipids with their headgroups," *Toxicology Research*, 7(3): 473–479.

[168] Brian C. Evans et al. (2019) "An anionic, endosome-escaping polymer to potentiate intracellular delivery of cationic peptides, biomacromolecules, and nanoparticles," *Nature Communications*, 10(5012): https://www.nature.com/articles/s41467-019-12906-y.

[169] Michael Looby and Peter Milligan (no date) *Dose – Exposure – Response Relationships: the Basis of Effective Dose-Regimen Selection*, https://www.ema.europa.eu/en/documents/presentation/presentation-dose-exposure-response-relationships-basis-effective-dose-regimen-selection-break-out_en.pdf.

[170] Ling-Yan Zhou et al. (2018) "Current Advances in Small Activating RNAs for Gene Therapy: Principles, Applications and Challenges," *Current Gene Therapy*, 18(3): 134-142.

[171] Tudor Emanuel Fertig et al. (2022) "Vaccine mRNA Can Be Detected in Blood at 15 Days Post-Vaccination," *Biomedicines*, 10(7): 10.3390/biomedicines10071538.

[172] Lael M. Yonker et al. (2023) "Circulating Spike Protein Detected in Post-COVID-19 mRNA Vaccine Myocarditis," *Circulation*, 147(11): 867-876.

[173] Jose Alfredo Samaniego Castruita et al. (2023) "SARS-CoV-2 spike mRNA vaccine sequences circulate in blood up to 28 days after COVID-19 vaccination," *Journal of Pathology, Microbiology and Immunology*, 131(3): 128-32.

[174] Michael Mörz (2022) "A Case Report: Multifocal Necrotizing Encephalitis and Myocarditis after BNT162b2 mRNA Vaccination against COVID-19," *Vaccines*, 10(10): 1651.

[175] Pfizer, "Annaliesa Anderson, Ph.D., Will Lead Pfizer's Vaccine Research & Development," 1 June 2022, https://www.pfizer.com/news/press-release/press-release-detail/annaliesa-anderson-phd-will-lead-pfizers-vaccine-research.

[176] Riley Griffin, "Pfizer Invests $470 Million to Develop Tech Behind Covid Shot," *Bloomberg*, 20 July 2022, https://www.bloomberg.com/news/articles/2022-07-20/pfizer-pfe-invests-470-million-to-build-covid-shot-tech-research-lab-near-nyc.

[177] Pfizer, "Pearl River, NY Site Statistics," no date, https://www.pfizer.com/pearl-river-new-york.

[178] Pfizer, "Single-plex Luminex Assay for Quantitation of IgG Antibodies to SARS-CoV-2 S1

Protein in Human Serum," Doc. No. VR-TM-10293, https://phmpt.org/wp-content/uploads/2023/04/125742_S1_M5_5314_vr-tm-10293.pdf.

[179] Biobide, "What is batch testing?," no date, https://blog.biobide.com/what-is-batch-testing.

[180] Paul Dabbar, "Running with the Speed of Science in the Race Against COVID-19," Department of Energy, 23 June 2020, https://www.energy.gov/articles/running-speed-science-race-against-covid-19.

[181] Thomas Gatliff, 13 October 2022, https://twitter.com/TGatliff/status/1580348039872798720.

[182] Annaliesa S. Anderson (2022) "A lightspeed approach to pandemic drug development," *Nature Medicine*, 28: 1538.

[183] Pfizer, "Annaliesa...," op. cit.

[184] Global Grand Challenges, "Production of a Transgenic Mosquito, as a Flying Syringe, to Deliver Protective Vaccine via Saliva," 1 October 2008, https://gcgh.grandchallenges.org/grant/production-transgenic-mosquito-flying-syringe-deliver-protective-vaccine-saliva.

[185] A screenshot of the tweet can be read here: Sarthak Dogra, "mRNA technology pioneer says Covid-19 vaccinated people can shed spike protein, Twitter says delete this," India Today, 31 May 2021, https://www.indiatoday.in/technology/news/story/mrna-technology-pioneer-says-covid-19-vaccinated-people-can-shed-spike-protein-twitter-says-delete-this-1809062-2021-05-31.

[186] WHO, "Boost for developing nations as mRNA technology hub moves to the next phase in South Africa," 20 April 2023, https://news.un.org/en/story/2023/04/1135907.

[187] Linda Geddes, "Machine versus virus: Deploying artificial intelligence against future pandemics," GAVI, 17 July 2023, https://www.gavi.org/vaccineswork/machine-versus-virus-deploying-artificial-intelligence-against-future-pandemics.

[188] Camille Bello, "Chinese tech giant Baidu is using AI to unlock better mRNA vaccines and cancer drugs. Here's how," EuroNews, 15 May 2023, https://www.euronews.com/next/2023/05/15/new-ai-algorithm-unlocks-most-stable-covid-vaccine-to-date-and-opens-door-to-new-cancer-dr.

[189] Healthcare Technology Report, "In a Surprising Turn, Moderna Will Work With China on mRNA Therapies," 14 August 2023, https://thehealthcaretechnologyreport.com/in-a-surprising-turn-moderna-will-work-with-china-on-mrna-therapies/.

[190] Roohi Mariam Peter, "mRNA vaccines: a promising future," Labiotech, 14 April 2023, https://www.labiotech.eu/in-depth/mrna-vaccines/.

[191] Department of Health and Aged Care (Australia), "mRNA therapies to stop heart disease," 26 July 2023, https://www.health.gov.au/news/mrna-therapies-to-stop-heart-disease.

[192] Jill Murphy, "EMA Aims to Develop Guideline for mRNA Vaccines," *BioPharm International*, 12 July 2023,

https://www.biopharminternational.com/view/ema-aims-to-develop-guideline-for-mrna-vaccines.
[193] William A. Haseltine, "How MRNA Could Reinvent Blood Stem Cell Transplant Preparations," *Forbes*, 15 August 2023, https://www.forbes.com/sites/williamhaseltine/2023/08/15/how-mrna-could-reinvent-blood-stem-cell-transplant-preparations/.

Index

9/11 41

ADEPT (see DARPA)
Anaphylaxis 96
Anderson, Annaliesa 108, 111
Appendicitis 37, 38
Arrhythmia 38
Arrhythmia death syndrome (see SADS)
Arteriosclerosis 66, 68
Autonomous Diagnostics to Enable Prevention and
Therapeutics (see DARPA)

Baidu 117
Baker Heart and Diabetes Institute 118
Bakewell, Joan 74
Bextra 46
Biden, Joe 17, 20, 47, 48
Bill and Melinda Gates Foundation 114
Bourla, Albert 48, 60-61, 63, 76
Brighton Collaboration 34
-CEPI 34
-SPEAC 34

Campanella, Olivia 85
Cancer 40, 66, 80, 83
CDC 47, 73, 74, 87

-Brighton Collaboration 34

-Maddie de Garay 14

Cellular Reprogramming 114

Centers for Disease Control and Prevention (see CDC)

CEPI 16, 17, 34, 116

-Brighton Collaboration 34

-WEF 34

Cerebral edema 67

Cerebrovascular disease 80

Choung, Captain James K. 42

Chronic pulmonary obstructive disease 66

Cincinnati Children's Hospital Medical Division 18

Cincinnati Children's Hospital Vaccine Research Center 10

Cincinnati Children's Hospital Vaccine Treatment and Evaluation Unit 10

Clotting 37, 38, 68

Coalition for Epidemic Preparedness Innovations (see CEPI)

CoronaVac 37

CSL 117

Cytochrome c oxidase 42

Dabbar, Paul 111

DARPA 40, 42

-ADEPT 43

-PREPARE 43

de Garay, Maddie 10-18, 27

de Garay, Patrick 10-18
de Garay, Stephanie 10-18
Defense Advanced Research Projects Agency (see DARPA)
Department of Energy 111
Department of Justice (see DOJ)
Diabetes 80
Diphtheria 62
DOJ 46, 49
Dormitzer, Philip 78
Doshi, Peter 21, 30

Emergency Use Authorization 20, 73, 88
European Commission 17

False Claims Act 22
Fauci, Dr. Anthony 48
FDA 47, 63, 66, 69, 72, 130n5
-Biologics License Application 52
-EUA 23, 63
-Maddie de Garay 14, 17
-Pfizer data 28, 30, 50-51, 58
Food and Drug Administration (see FDA)
Fort Detrick 40, 42, 44
Fox News 15
Frenck, Robert 14, 17-18

Gates, Bill 16-17, 60

Gatliff, Thomas 111
GAVI 16, 17, 116
Georgia Institute of Technology 44
Grand Challenges in Global Health 114
Gruber, Marion 47

Haemophilus influenza type-B 62
Hepatitis B 61-62
Hepatitis C 104
Hepatotoxicity 82, 100
Herpes zoster 37
HIV 116
Hotez, Peter 20

Icon 22, 24, 26
Interstitial nephritis 81
Isch(a)emic stroke 38
Isc(a)emic heart disease 80
Israel Democracy Institute 78-79
Ivermectin 76-77

Jackson, Brook 12, 21-26
Janssen 36
Johnson, Boris 17

Kotler, Dr. Sarah 84
Krause, Philip 47

Lassa virus 44, 117
Lipid nanoparticles (see LNPs)
LNPs 35, 98, 101
Lymphadenopathy 37

Malone, Dr. Robert
Matsuoka, Hiroyuki 114
McAnallen, Cormac 74
Merkel, Angela 17
Merriam-Webster 50
Mineo, Gosia 72
Moderna 19, 31, 38, 41, 44, 51, 117, 135n39
mRNA 12, 20, 34-45, 48, 51, 61, 99, 102, 104-06, 111, 114-19
Myocardial infarction 38
Myocarditis 37, 66, 69, 71, 96

National Health and Medical Research Council 118
National Institute of Allergy and Infectious Diseases 48
National Institutes of Health (see NIH)
Nephropathy 81
NIH
-Maddie de Garay 14
Nipah virus 117
Nuremberg Code 15

O'Shaughnessy, Jacqueline 72
Office for Health Improvement and Disparities 80

Oxford-AstraZeneca 19

Paresthesia 14
Paxlovid 76
PEGylated 99
Pericarditis 92, 96
Periods 71
Pertussis 62
Pharmacia & Upjohn 46
Pittman, Judge Mark 11, 49
Polyethylene glycol (see PEGylated)
PReemptive Expression of Protective Alleles and
Response Elements (see DARPA)
PREPARE (see DARPA)
Prostaglandin E2 42
Public Health and Medical Professionals for
Transparency 48
Pulmonary embolism 38

SADS 74-75
Safety Platform for Emergency Vaccines 34
Sanofi 117
Santangelo, Dr. Phil 44
Second World War (see WWII)
Sepsis 66
Settembre, Ethan 118
Shwartz Altshuler, Tehilla 78-79
Sputnik V 19
Stroke 38

See also ischemic stroke.
Sudden adult death syndrome (see SADS)
Swelling 10, 102
-Cerebral edema 67
-Lymph nodes 11
-Necrotising encephalitis 105

Tachycardia 10
Tetanus
ThermoFisher 109
Thromboembolism (see clotting)
Thrombosis (see clotting)
Tinnitus 11
Trump, Donald 20, 48

United Nations (see UN)
US Army Medical Research and Development Command 44

Vaccine Adverse Event Reporting System (see VAERS)
Vaccine Alliance (see GAVI)
VAERS 14, 93
Venatavia 12, 21-26

Warren, Luigi 114
Wellcome Trust 17
Weng, Xiaowei 118
Whitehead, Dr. Kathryn A. 43

WHO 15
-Bill Gates 16
-CEPI 16, 17
-Corruption 16, 116
-GAVI 16, 17
World Economic Forum 16, 60-61, 116
World Health Organization (see WHO)
WWII 41